Dizziness

A Johns Hopkins Press Health Book

Dizziness

Why You Feel Dizzy
and
What Will Help You
Feel Better

GREGORY T. WHITMAN, MD
and ROBERT W. BALOH, MD

Johns Hopkins University Press • *Baltimore*

Note to the Reader: This book is not meant to substitute for medical care of people with dizziness, and treatment should not be based solely on its contents. Instead, treatment must be developed in a dialogue between the individual and his or her physician. Our book has been written to help with that dialogue.

Drug dosage: The authors and publisher have made reasonable efforts to determine that the selection of drugs discussed in this text conform to the practices of the general medical community. The medications described do not necessarily have specific approval by the US Food and Drug Administration for use in the diseases for which they are recommended. In view of ongoing research, changes in governmental regulation, and the constant flow of information relating to drug therapy and drug reactions, the reader is urged to check the package insert of each drug for any change in indications and dosage and for warnings and precautions. This is particularly important when the recommended agent is a new and/or infrequently used drug.

© 2016 Johns Hopkins University Press
All rights reserved. Published 2016
Printed in the United States of America on acid-free paper
9 8 7 6 5 4 3 2

Johns Hopkins University Press
2715 North Charles Street
Baltimore, Maryland 21218-4363
www.press.jhu.edu

Library of Congress Cataloging-in-Publication Data

Names: Whitman, Gregory T., 1966– author. | Baloh, Robert W. (Robert William), 1942– author.
Title: Dizziness : why you feel dizzy and what will help you feel better / Gregory T. Whitman, MD, and Robert W. Baloh, MD.
Description: Baltimore : Johns Hopkins University Press, 2016. | Series: A Johns Hopkins Press health book | Includes bibliographical references and index.
Identifiers: LCCN 2016002111 | ISBN 9781421420899 (hardback) | ISBN 9781421420905 (paperback) | ISBN 9781421420912 (electronic)
Subjects: LCSH: Dizziness. | Vertigo. | Vestibular apparatus—Diseases. | BISAC: HEALTH & FITNESS / General. | MEDICAL / Neurology. | HEALTH & FITNESS / Diseases / General.
Classification: LCC RB150.V4 W45 2016 | DDC 616.8/41—dc23
LC record available at https://lccn.loc.gov/2016002111

A catalog record for this book is available from the British Library.

Special discounts are available for bulk purchases of this book. For more information, please contact Special Sales at 410-516-6936 or specialsales@press.jhu.edu.

Johns Hopkins University Press uses environmentally friendly book materials, including recycled text paper that is composed of at least 30 percent post-consumer waste, whenever possible.

To our wives, Sally and Grace, who provided the inspiration, and to our dizzy patients—you have taught us more than any book

Contents

Preface

You should read this book if you are dizzy, if you are lightheaded, if your world seems to move when it shouldn't, or if you are off balance and have fallen. The authors of this book specialize in taking care of people with **dizziness** and **imbalance** and they understand how distressing these symptoms can be. (Words appearing in boldface type are defined in the glossary at the back of the book.)

People with dizziness tell us we are their "last hope." We believe that's an overstatement, but it captures the way many dizzy people feel. The good news is there are always things we can do for people with dizziness. This untapped therapeutic potential is what gets us into the clinic on days we see patients. Our clinics and those like them go by a variety of names. Sometimes our specialty is called otoneurology (a term that is used a lot in Boston) or neuro-otology (a hyphenated term that has been sanctioned by the American Academy of Neurology), or neurotology (used at the University of California at Los Angeles, though not without slight confusion because there is also a surgical specialty called neurotology, which is a branch of otolaryngology). Whatever you call it, our specialty involves making a diagnosis and prescribing treatment for people with dizziness and imbalance.

Most people with dizziness will be treated first by a generalist, such as a doctor trained in internal medicine, family practice, or emergency medicine. In many cases, the generalist's approaches work well. But many generalists go only so far with dizziness. They have a few reasonable responses to dizziness in their toolbox. When these do not work, many refer dizzy people to clinics like ours, at least in regions of the country where such clinics exist. We hope this book will fill a need for people who do not have access to a dizziness specialist and enhance care for those who do have such access.

In this book, we start from the assumption that the reader would like to know how the best doctors make a diagnosis. We base this assumption on our experience with many thousands of patients. Many people with dizziness have seen multiple doctors, and none of these doctors has been able to make a clear diagnosis. The reader may have nothing to go on, other than his or her symptoms. Therefore, we focus on symptoms. We have divided the book into parts, each of which addresses a particular class of symptoms. Within each such part, we discuss specific diseases: how they are defined and diagnosed, how doctors and scientists understand the disease, and the best approaches to treatment. Childhood dizziness could be the focus of a whole book and as such is beyond the scope of the present volume, though many of our comments are applicable to children as well as adults.

How did we decide which diseases to include? We admit that this was a challenge. We apologize in advance to those for whom we have omitted something important. An essential problem is that almost every disease can cause dizziness. We must always therefore be on the alert for a serious disease presenting as "dizziness." Some examples are stroke, transient ischemic attacks (TIAs), multiple sclerosis, and brain tumors. The doctor who cares for people with dizziness must have a solid grasp of general medicine. Despite this array of possibilities, though, the vast majority of people who come to our dizziness clinics have something not so serious, though even a short-lived problem can make the affected person feel very sick for a period of time.

Medical students are taught to concentrate on the common causes of symptoms. The focus on the common is encapsulated by the old saying that when one hears hoofbeats, it is best to think of horses, not of zebras. We will tell you about the most common problems experienced by our patients. In addition, we will identify so-called red flags—symptoms that suggest the possibility that something more serious is going on. We also give the reader some ideas about how we recognize that we are dealing with a less common disorder—a zebra and not a horse.

With respect to the common, one might ask: why focus on our own clinics at UCLA- and Harvard-affiliated hospitals? Isn't that asking for bias? Do our clinics reflect the experience of people in general? We thought about this. There are two answers. We are familiar with dizziness specialty clinics across the United States and overseas. In general, dizziness clinics that are staffed by neurologists are remarkably similar. The mixture of diagnoses does not differ drastically from one to the next. If you are seen by a neurology clinic that specializes in dizziness, you can pretty much bet that the other people in the waiting room, and quite possibly you, will experience issues discussed in this book. The second reason for our choice of diseases is that these are the ones we know best. The problems described in this book are problems we have seen hundreds, or in some cases thousands, of times. We feel we can most authoritatively comment on those disorders with which we have the greatest experience. Considering how common dizziness is in general, we think that by simply telling stories about what we have personally seen on the front lines, we may be able to do some good.

In addition to common problems, we also focus on serious ones. Many of our patients want to know if there is something serious going on. To some degree, seriousness is in the eye of the beholder. It is always unnerving to hear a medical intern describe a patient in the intensive care unit as doing "fine" or "great." Obviously, a person wouldn't be in the ICU if they were doing great. To some extent, seriousness is a matter of perspective. Sometimes, disorders that doctors consider to be serious differ from those that patients consider to be serious. In any event, the question, "Is this something serious?" is a major source of anxiety for patients, their families, friends, and coworkers. Therefore, we have suggested some approaches to the identification of serious disorders.

In the detection of potentially serious problems, one strategy experienced doctors use is to pay careful attention to any symptoms that deviate from the expected. If something doesn't make sense, one should be a little worried. To use this strategy, one must first have a firm grip on what the most common disorders are supposed to look like. Only then can one recognize patterns that deviate from the norm. In other words, one must be alert for atypical patterns. This is a skill that takes years to develop, and it is one of the reasons dizzy people sometimes need help from doctors.

Many readers of this book will be seeking answers on how to get to a clear diagnosis. While we cannot make the reader the equal of an experienced doctor, we can probably teach you how to use some pattern recognition to your advantage. The awesome power of pattern recognition is well known to neurologists. A classic example is Parkinson disease. Neurologists can recognize Parkinson disease within a few seconds. The overall slowing of movement, including facial expressions, a tendency to not blink as much as normal and to not shift in a chair as much as one would expect, a slight restlessness of a limb, a slightly stooped posture, and other cues of which we probably are not aware all ring bells for the average neurologist. They indicate the likelihood of Parkinson disease. Pattern recognition, though, extends well beyond diagnosis of Parkinson disease. The common disorders that cause dizziness have stereotyped patterns. These can usually be recognized within a couple minutes of speaking with a person.

Some doctors have a natural talent for pattern recognition. The nineteenth-century French neurologist Jean-Martin Charcot added much to our specialty of neurology. Charcot was a painter. There is little doubt that he used his artistic vision to his advantage in understanding his patients. Similarly, Leonardo da Vinci is best known as an artist and inventor. But he contributed to the medical field through his paintings of human anatomy. His talent for using vision—in brief, his ability to see like an artist—is something many people have. In fact, we believe that any person who takes the trouble to look carefully has the potential to see like an artist. In doing so, almost anyone can help friends and family in the process of getting a diagnosis. Family members or friends around a person with dizziness, if they take the trouble to pay attention to the affected individual, can help contribute to a rapid and correct diagnosis. In this book, we hope to recruit and nurture such observers. We hope to increase the interested individual's powers of observation. After reading this book, it should be possible for someone to recognize the correct diagnosis in a great many circumstances—not all, but many.

In practice, doctors often explicitly or implicitly look for so-called red flags—particular well-accepted indicators of serious disease. We describe some red flags in this book. When symptoms expressed in the dizziness clinic are out of the norm—when they are atypical—it's usually a red flag. Because most diseases can cause dizziness, it would be completely logical to write a book on dizziness that covers all of general medicine. We aren't going to try to do that. It isn't possible in a small book. We do, however, hope to convey an appreciation of the large spectrum of possibilities when a person feels dizzy.

In each section on a particular disease category, we address best treatment. We provide information about critical actions a person can take to help alleviate symptoms without the need for any prescribed medicine, injections, or surgery. These actions might be described as self-help. Because self-help can only go so far, we suggest ways in which a person can most effectively partner with doctors.

Dizziness is so overwhelmingly common that nearly everyone will experience it. Dizziness and imbalance have major implications for important aspects of life: productivity on the job, participating in family and friendship, ability to drive, the risk for falls and injuries, and at a fundamental level, one's identity and sense of self. People are mostly unaware of the body's remarkable system for maintaining balance until something goes wrong. Then, all of a sudden, your world is turned upside down, moves sideways or rocks like a boat on rough seas, and you can't stand, walk, or really do anything normally. It is for these people that we wrote this book, in the hope that their days may be made more pleasant and productive.

Dizziness

Introduction

I find it hard to recognize some relatives of ours, like the rotifer, the
sycamore, iguanas, and sea stars.

—*They Might Be Giants*

In their song about evolution, "My Brother the Ape," the
American rock band They Might Be Giants observed that
humans are relatives of trees, lizards, and starfish. But can
one really make a comparison between a tree and a person?
Indeed, we have a lot in common with plants. Like plants,
people are made of **cells**. The cells are made up of proteins.
One aspect shared by all living things is that we evolved in a
gravitational field owing to the immense mass of the Earth.

A feature all living organisms share is the ability to orient
with respect to gravity, to tell up from down. Even the most
basic single-cell forms of life such as bacteria and algae "detect" the pull of gravity, probably by differences in density at
different parts of the cell. If the stems of plants are placed flat,
they will grow faster on the upper side and turn upward as
heavier substances gather in greater concentration on the
lower side of the stem. Specialized organs used to sense
gravity are already seen in primitive animals such as jelly-
fish, which appeared more than 600 million years ago on the

evolutionary time scale. In these animals, a pouch filled with seawater, the otocyst, contains tiny stones, or "liths," whose density is much greater than the surrounding fluid. Gravity causes these tiny stones to rest their weight on specialized sensing cells in the walls of the pouch, allowing the animals to regulate their position in space.

This primitive otocyst is the forerunner of the inner ear in more advanced animals. In his famous work, *On the Origin of Species*, Charles Darwin used a tree to illustrate the concept of evolution. On this so-called tree of life, the primitive otocyst is located at the main trunk while the inner ears of the most advanced animals are located at the most peripheral branches.

In early fish, the pouch previously open to the outside becomes closed and is filled with fluid secreted by cells in the wall of the cyst. The otolith organ remains relatively unchanged, but the other parts of the inner ear—the sensors for rotation of the head, the **semicircular canals**, and the sensors for hearing, the cochlea—develop later but are already present in modern fish that evolved about 100 million years ago. The vestibular part of the inner ear, the **otolith organs** and the semicircular canals, are relatively unchanged from fish to primates, including humans.

In its simplest form, dizziness is a problem with orientation, a feeling of disorientation. Since the inner ear is a key organ for providing the brain with orientating information, damage to the inner ear can cause dizziness. Although it seems intuitive now, it is remarkable how long it took the medical community to understand this simple concept. The symptom of dizziness had been recognized for several thousand years, but it wasn't until the pioneering work of Prosper Ménière in the mid nineteenth century that it was appreciated that dizziness could originate from damage to the inner ear. Prior to that time, a patient with dizziness was said to have "cerebral congestion," a condition resulting from excessive blood filling the brain. Bloodletting and leeches to relieve the congestion were the treatments of choice.

Ménière, who directed a Paris institute for people who could neither hear nor speak, made the simple observation that patients who developed sudden deafness, such as occurred after being shot in the ear with an arrow, also had severe dizziness and **disequilibrium**. He concluded that parts of the inner ear must be important for orientation and balance, in addition to hearing. Although detailed anatomy of the inner ear had been described as early as the mid-sixteenth century, the vestibular part of the inner ear was thought to be involved in hearing, not balance. For example, the semicircular canals were thought to be important for identifying the location of sounds in space, not for sensing motion of the head in space. Based on his experience, Ménière pointed out that patients with acute hearing loss and dizziness usually had a benign course and that aggressive treatments such as bleeding were more dangerous than the underlying disorder. Knowing what we know today, this seems straightforward common sense, but in the middle of the nineteenth century it was considered heretical.

One obvious difference between people and plants is mobility. The central nature of mobility to human beings is reflected in our languages. People "go" for it. They "run" organizations. If something is easy, it is said to be a "walk in the park." Mobility is a core aspect of the human experience. Loss of mobility is devastating. And it is hard to think of any disease that cannot affect balance if the disease is severe enough.

For older people in particular, the ability to balance and walk is a critical survival skill. The US Centers for Disease Control and Prevention describe falls as the leading cause of injuries, both fatal and nonfatal. And falls take away independence.

All experienced doctors have met an older person who was injured in a fall and as a result wound up in a nursing home for a prolonged period, or even permanently. Mobility defines us, and loss of mobility is a significant cause of loss of independence and shortened life-span.

Those who specialize in dizziness and balance inevitably have an interest in the human brain. Can we gain insight into the basis for human mobility by studying the anatomy of the brain? If you watch late-night infomercials on television, you might get the idea that scientists have it all figured out. They know what parts of the brain are responsible for each human function.

Patients often ask us to explain how a particular disease works, in terms of parts of the brain and their connections. We sometimes attempt to do this, using a pencil and paper, a picture, or a 3D model. This is an interesting but less than satisfying exercise. When you specialize in dizziness and balance, you quickly realize that balance involves the whole brain and its trillions of connections. Understanding dizziness is more complicated than understanding some other neurological disorders, such as carpal tunnel syndrome. In carpal tunnel syndrome, the median nerve, compressed in the carpal tunnel of the wrist, stops working correctly, resulting in numbness and weakness. Normal balance, in contrast, depends on almost the entire brain. Balance is inherently all about integrating and using many types of information from all of the senses with memory, planning, and other supportive functions.

There are two reasons we teach anatomy to medical students. At a superficial level—the level that, to paraphrase Yogi Berra, you can see just by looking with your eyes—anatomy helps greatly with diagnosis, as we will explain. You can see the wrist, and you can press over the median nerve and ask the patient if she feels a tingling sensation. If the answer is yes, then she has carpal tunnel syndrome. The kind of anatomy you can see with your eyes and feel on examination turns out to help greatly with diagnosis. The second reason we teach anatomy to medical students is that it is an entrée into the world of scientific research, a path only a minority of medical students will follow. Yet we need these researchers to make future medical discoveries. We should not delude ourselves, though, into thinking that we can fully explain balance by drawing a picture of anatomic pathways on a piece of paper. At the level of the individual cells of the brain—the **neurons** and **glial cells**—it is less clear that we can apply anatomic knowledge to treatment of patients.

As a result, the pragmatic dizziness specialist is more interested in function than in structure. The reason is simple. The brain is too complicated to allow a detailed analysis of its circuits. Realistically, we do not know the wiring diagram of anything close to a human brain. At the time of this writing, scientists remain excited about the wiring diagram for the nervous system of *Caenorhabditis elegans*, a tiny worm that lives in the soil and survives on a hearty diet of bacteria. That scientists are thrilled by the brain wiring of this worm—302 neurons, give or take—highlights our ignorance about how the nervous system works in humans.

The modern study of the detailed wiring diagrams of circuits in the brain is sometimes called connectomics. A leading connectomics group—the lab of Dr. Sebastian Seung at the Massachusetts Institute of Technology—has focused lately on mapping the retina. Dr. Seung has also done advanced scientific work on the physiology of the inner ear balance system and its connections in the brain and continues to work in this area. In the past few years, though, his group has published articles in a top scientific journal describing the connections of cells in the retina. At the moment, studying selected cells in the retina is exactly the type of small connectomics project that can succeed. Mapping the whole brain or even a small part of the brain with an anatomical name such as "the hippocampus" represents a worthy goal that for the moment remains out of reach. We'll get there, but not this year.

Even Dr. Seung's recent, limited map of a small part of the retinal wiring diagram could not have been completed without relying on "crowdsourcing" of more than 2,000 citizen neuroscientists who helped with the project. This tour de force of human effort was required, in addition to some of the best minds and computers available at MIT, in order to achieve just a small piece of the wiring diagram for a small patch of tissue in a single layer of the retina. So we have a long way to go. We do not understand the wiring diagram of the brain in enough detail to fully explain balance.

On the other hand, gross anatomy—the kind that you can see just by looking—is of great use to the doctor. Neurologists, in particular, rely on anatomic localization, a process of listening to and examining a person that leads to localizations—sites at which the doctor thinks there is disease. Anatomic localization allows us and other neurologists to rapidly determine, in broad terms, where the problem is. We ask ourselves, "Could the problem be in the peripheral nerves located in the legs? Or in the carpal tunnel? Or in the brain? If the problem is in the brain, is it located on the left side or the right side, the front or back, or one of the deep structures such as the brain stem or cerebellum?" Once a neurologist knows "where" the problem is, it is easier to determine "what" the problem is. The list of possible diagnoses— the **differential diagnosis**—is narrowed. For example, the list of possible causes of a slow degeneration of nerves in the legs differs greatly from causes of inability to speak.

Dizziness specialists spend much of their time measuring function. How variable is a person's step length? How many steps, heel to toe, can a person take before taking a side step? What's the maximum eye speed that can be induced by turning a person to the right and left? What's the most miniscule acceleration a person can detect in darkness? Outside of a few brave anatomists, most people in our field of balance are primarily interested in function. To us, this means **physiology**— the ways the nervous system *functions*, rather than the *structure* of the nervous system (which is the anatomy). Many of the phenomena that a scientist would call physiology are reflected in variation of some observable entity with time, such as change in eye position with time, or the rate of contraction of muscles on one side of the face compared to the other. Your doctor can see such changes on a physical examination. In particular, the classical neurological examination that all neurology trainees learn is well suited to recognize characteristic patterns associated with dizziness or disturbances of balance. (The abnormalities a doctor can see on a neurological examination are described in later chapters of this book.)

Medical students are traditionally encouraged to "read about your patients." It's infinitely easier to remember the details of a real person than to memorize long lists of unrelated facts. Accordingly, our book includes stories. These stories will help you understand key principles. These are true stories, though some details have been changed to protect our patients' privacy. We have intentionally picked some case examples with bad outcomes since it is possible to learn a great deal from mistakes. Some of our stories may seem cynical. These reflect our frustration with how our health care system treats dizzy patients. Indeed, we decided to write this book because of the way dizzy patients are treated in the health care system.

We have aimed to include in each chapter some information about the history of neurology as it pertains to the subject of dizziness, including some of the most famous contributors to our specialty. This is not only because both authors have an interest in the historical aspects of our profession but also because we feel that the reader—by following a little of the path along which ideas were developed—will gain insight into modern principles.

As individual doctors working in our clinics, we can probably each only personally treat, at most, a couple thousand people per year. Through this book, we hope to teach some principles that will allow anyone to better understand dizziness and balance. For each dizziness problem we provide a survey of the types of symptoms and physical findings expected. We discuss self-help strategies and self-help interventions for the purpose of speeding the processes of diagnosis and healing, and we describe how you can partner with your doctors to get the best care. We cannot teach readers enough to diagnose themselves fully. However, we are hopeful that by focusing on problems we see frequently, and by explaining them in plain English, we will allow readers to do almost as well as doctors in the *initial* approach to dizziness and imbalance.

Before launching into a discussion of the disorders that cause dizziness and imbalance, it is important to clarify some of the vocabulary we use (and the glossary at the end of the book can remind readers of definitions when needed). One of the most important words is **vertigo**. Vertigo may be defined as a feeling that either you or your environment is moving or spinning, when in fact nothing of the sort is happening. Vertigo is suggestive, although not proof, that there is a problem in the **vestibular system**, the balance-related sensory structures of the inner ear (the otolith organs and semicircular canals), combined with their connections in the brain.

Dizziness is a broad catch-all term. It encompasses vertigo but also a range of other abnormal sensations, including lightheadedness or faintness. When dizziness specialists use the term "vertigo," there is often an implication that the problem resides in the vestibular system. When they use the term "dizziness," all bets are off. The problem could be just about anything. The reader should realize that almost any disorder, and all medications, have made somebody dizzy. However, as we will see, most of the common causes of dizziness can be easily recognized and successfully treated.

Equally important to recognize are symptoms described by the terms "disequilibrium" and "imbalance." These terms mean someone has difficulty controlling body position, such as while walking. Disequilibrium and imbalance do not imply a particular anatomic localization such as the vestibular system. Indeed, almost any **central nervous system** problem—in the brain or spinal cord—is likely to cause imbalance in some individuals. For practical purposes, disorders that involve imbalance also essentially always cause an abnormality of gait, affect mobility, and increase the risk of falling.

Another term important to the understanding of dizziness is **nystagmus**. Nystagmus means repetitive jerking of the eyes, usually in a pattern that is extremely useful for diagnosis. Show us a video of the nystagmus, and we can probably tell you where it is coming from. Most nystagmus is what's called jerk nystagmus, in which there is a well-defined slow drift in one direction, called a slow phase, followed by a quick jerk in the opposite direction. This pattern repeats itself, giving the appearance of eyes jerking in a particular direction. By convention, nystagmus is named by the direction of the fast phase. If the slow phases are toward the person's right side and the quick jerks are toward the person's left side, we call it left-beating nystagmus.

Ask doctors what one needs to know to diagnose a dizzy person, and many will answer that one must first decide whether the problem is peripheral or central. A peripheral vestibular problem is caused by problems of the inner ear or the vestibular nerve (the nerve that projects from the inner ear to the brain). A central vestibular problem involves the brain. The **peripheral vestibular system** consists of the portions of the inner ear that support balance function, plus the vestibular nerve. **Central vestibular pathways** are mainly located in the brain stem and **cerebellum,** but there are vestibular-related pathways throughout the brain. Many disorders involve both peripheral and central deficits, but neurologists still find that it is worth considering where the most critical aspects of the problem are located. This often speeds up diagnosis and helps them select treatments that are most likely to be effective.

One of the discussions we often have in clinic is about the meaning of the word "ear." Often, we think of the ear as one entity, but it really isn't. The ear has three distinct structures, the terms for which all have the word "ear" in their name: the **external ear,** the **middle ear,** and the **inner ear** (figure 1). When most people think of the ear, they picture the earlobe, and maybe the external auditory canal, where water can enter during swimming. Earwax (cerumen) occurs in the external auditory canal. In practical terms, the external auditory canal contributes nothing to balance, disturbances of balance, or dizziness. People often wonder whether cerumen is a cause of dizziness, and the answer is basically no. If there is a lot of cerumen present, it can be a little distracting and may affect hearing. However, cerumen is normal. It protects the ear and, if present in small amounts, should not be removed. At the in-

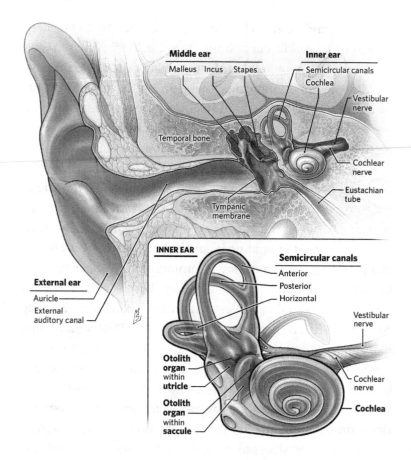

Figure 1 Cross-section of the ear showing the external ear, middle ear, and inner ear. Inset shows the inner ear in greater detail. Terms are defined in the text and glossary.

side end of the external auditory canal, one encounters the tympanic membrane, also known as the eardrum.

Beyond the eardrum is the middle ear. A doctor can sometimes look through the eardrum to see the middle ear with an otoscope and can then say things like, "I can see that you have fluid" or "I can see that you have an ear infection." When doctors say these things, they are referring to what they can see in the middle ear. There is a lot of confusion, in our field, between the middle ear and the inner ear. Many children have experienced a middle ear infection, also called otitis media. Middle ear infections cause ear pain but in general do not cause dizziness. Middle ear infections rarely spread to the inner ear, particularly in the current "antibiotic era," when effective antibiotics can clear the infection.

The middle ear has little to do with balance. There is a tube from the middle ear to the back of the throat called the Eustachian tube. The Eustachian tube is important for equalizing pressure between the outside world and the middle ear, such as during ascent or landing in an airplane. Blockage of the Eustachian tube is an extremely common cause of ear fullness but not a common cause of dizziness. People with dizziness and ear fullness due to Eustachian tube blockage typically have two different things going on—the Eustachian tube blockage and the dizziness. These need to be treated separately. Eustachian tube blockage is beyond the scope of this book, except to say that it is sometimes treated with nasal rinses and nasal sprays, allergy medicines, and other interventions aimed at opening up the Eustachian tube and restoring the ability to equalize pressure. These treatments will seldom help with dizziness. In the normal middle ear, three tiny bones (the malleus, incus, and stapes) conduct sound. The stapes vibrates the oval window between the middle ear and the inner ear. The oval window sends vibrations into the inner ear that the brain ultimately perceives as sound. This book does not focus on hearing, which is a fascinating function of the inner ear that is more or less distinct from balance function.

The inner ear, where the balance organs are located, is far removed from the outside world. It is encased in bone next to the brain. The inner ear cannot be seen on a physical examination. Moreover, the inner ear is not well visualized on current **MRI scans** because of its small size (the size of the tip of your little finger).

With that brief introduction to vocabulary and anatomy, off we go to the dizziness clinic. Additional anatomy and physiology are introduced along the way, where appropriate, to increase the reader's understanding.

PART I DIZZY SPELLS THAT OCCUR WITH A CHANGE IN POSITION

CHAPTER 1

Benign Paroxysmal Positional Vertigo

Within a few seconds of changing position (lying down, turning in bed, or bending the head backward while sitting or standing), you feel a wave of vertigo that typically lasts 10 to 30 seconds. You may also feel dizzy all day long. But this is a different, milder kind of dizziness, typically a motion sickness.

Vertigo that is triggered by a change in head position is called positional vertigo. Benign paroxysmal positional vertigo (BPPV) is the most common type of positional vertigo, but it is not the only type. BPPV is a distinct diagnosis with known cause (see below), while positional vertigo is a symptom with many causes. After lying down or turning over in bed, a person with BPPV feels that the world seems to move or spin. In some cases, a person with BPPV may feel that an object in the room, such as an alarm clock, appears to jump up and down rhythmically.

As noted in the introduction, there are two types of motion sensors in the inner ear: the otolith organs, which are sensitive to gravity, and the semicircular canals, which are sensitive to rotation of the head. BPPV occurs when the tiny stones, "otoliths" (also called **otoconia**), sitting on top of the otolith organs become dislodged and fall into one of the semicircular canals. Normally, the semicircular canals are not sensitive to changes in the direction of gravity that occur with head position change, but when the "heavy" otolith debris enters a semicircular canal, the canal becomes sensitive to gravity. Movement of debris within a semicircular canal activates the sensors in the semicircular canal, sending a signal to the brain to indicate that you are spinning in the plane of the canal. The vertigo sensation is brief (seconds) since the debris stops moving when it settles. The debris almost always gets trapped in the posterior semicircular canal because of its position in the inner ear.

That BPPV was a benign disorder originating from the inner ear was first reported in the early 1950s. Initially, BPPV was thought to result from damage to the otolith organs since they were the ones sensitive to gravity. However, doctors performing postmortem studies of people who had had BPPV noticed otolith debris in the semicircular canals. They proposed the theory of "canal lithiasis" (stones in the canal). This term is ordinarily written in a shortened form as **canalithiasis**. Based on this theory, in the late 1980s, John Epley, an otolaryngologist in Oregon, introduced a simple positioning maneuver designed to "roll" the otolith debris out of the canal (now called the **Epley maneuver**), curing positional vertigo.

For several years after the Epley maneuver was introduced, there was great skepticism within the medical community regarding its effectiveness. Such simple cures just don't exist in medicine. By the turn of the century, a few skeptics remained, but most had jumped on the bandwagon after seeing how dramatic the cure can be. The American Academy of Neurology and the American Academy of Otolaryngology and Head and Neck Surgery recently published position papers strongly endorsing the Epley treatment maneuver for BPPV. Put simply, it works! (See "What Is the Best Treatment for BPPV?" later in this chapter.)

What happens to the debris once it is out of the canal and back into the chamber containing the otolith organ (called the **utricle**)? It may continue to float around and later reenter the canal, it may dissolve in the inner ear fluid, or it may be incorporated into the inner ear membrane. We know relatively little about how the debris is eliminated although the calcium concentration of the inner ear fluid seems to affect whether the debris will dissolve.

So we know that otolith debris that is rich in calcium becomes dislodged from the otolith organ and causes BPPV. But why does it become dislodged? One obvious cause is a blow to the head that is forceful enough to dislodge the otoliths. BPPV is common after major head injuries. The most common risk factor for developing BPPV, however, is normal aging. The otoliths are less tightly bound to the underlying sensory cells as we age. Approximately one in five people in their eighties will develop BPPV. By contrast, when we see BPPV in young subjects, there is a good likelihood that they already have, or will at some point develop, **migraine** headaches. How migraine predisposes to BPPV is completely unknown.

Along with bones and teeth, otoliths are heavily invested with calcium. Might we learn something about BPPV from what we know about the common bone disease osteoporosis? In fact, people with BPPV appear to be at risk for osteoporosis. We don't know why. But when we see a person with BPPV, we encourage follow up with a primary care doctor for prevention or treatment of osteoporosis. It has also recently been found that people with BPPV are at risk for vitamin D deficiency. It would be nice to be able to conclude that we can decrease the likelihood of a recurrence of BPPV just by giving vitamin D. Unfortunately, we can't say that. What we can recommend is for people with BPPV to have a blood test of the 25-hydroxy-vitamin D level. At present, a clinical trial is under way in Korea to determine whether BPPV recurrences can be decreased in frequency or prevented by taking vitamin D and calcium.

Typical Symptoms of BPPV

People with BPPV have distinct, easily recognizable symptoms. If you have BPPV, one or more of the following will occur. You will wake up dizzy. Or dizziness will occur when lying down or turning over in bed. Or dizziness may be triggered by looking up while sitting or standing, such as reaching for something on a top shelf (often called "top shelf vertigo"). Most people with BPPV will have more than one of these symptoms. Other than BPPV there are few medical conditions that cause a person to experience spinning that is triggered by lying down. Therefore, we always ask about whether dizziness is triggered by lying down.

You may have heard that BPPV can occur after sitting up from a lying-down position. This is absolutely true. However, many things other than BPPV also cause dizziness upon sitting up. One of the goals of this book is to teach you about symptoms that are highly sensitive (meaning one is unlikely to miss the diagnosis if one requires the symptom for diagnosis) and highly specific (meaning that one will not falsely label a person as having the diagnosis as a result of requiring the symptom for diagnosis). Sensitive findings are good because they can help a doctor avoid overlooking a diagnosis. Specific findings are good because they lead to one and only one diagnosis. Dizziness on sitting up is a sensitive symptom: most people with BPPV do experience it. However, it is nonspecific; relying on this symptom alone may lead one to falsely conclude that a person has BPPV instead of a different but correct diagnosis. The concept of specificity is critical for correct diagnosis. With respect to a physical finding on examination or diagnostic test, **specificity** measures how often normal people will be labeled as such. A finding with a low specificity, also called a nonspecific finding, often incorrectly flags perfectly normal people as abnormal. Nonspecific findings should be noted but also must be taken with a grain of salt. If your doctor refers to a test result or exam finding as nonspecific, it means that it should not be used as the primary argument for a diagnosis.

People with BPPV may also have difficulty describing feelings of dizziness that linger throughout the day. This lingering sensation may lead people to conclude that their condition can't be BPPV because BPPV only lasts for a few seconds when, for example, the person lies down. However, the dramatic spinning spells only occur with position change.

CASE EXAMPLE: What Can Go Wrong?

Ellen, an 80-year-old retired librarian, reached up toward the ceiling to place a folder on the top shelf of a closet. An unseen force began to pull her backward. She nearly fell. Confined in a narrow hallway, she placed a palm against the nearby wall. "What was that?" she thought. She walked slowly to the living room and sat on the couch. She decided to lie down, thinking this might make her feel better, but doing so triggered an even more violent attack of vertigo. She felt ill, as though she might vomit. Her husband called their primary care doctor. The staff agreed to fit her in. She didn't want to wait several hours to be seen in an emergency room. But was she making the right decision? Was she having a **stroke**?

At the office, her doctor was warm and friendly. He listened attentively. He checked her heart and lungs. "I know what this is," he said. "It's vertigo. I am going to write you a prescription for meclizine, an antihistamine that acts on the brain to suppress vertigo and nausea. It should pass in a few days." She was left with many questions. What did he mean by vertigo? How does he know I'm not having a stroke? But the doctor was busy and moved on to the next patient.

Back at home she decided to rest. She tried to lie down in bed, and the world spun violently—a nauseating tornado of motion. Slight movements caused the tornado to occur again. Something was wrong. Had her doctor made an error? Her husband called the paramedics, who rushed her to an emergency room. A **CT scan** of the head showed nothing, apart from her normal-appearing brain. After consultation with the emergency room doctors, she was admitted to the hospital, primarily to be sure she hadn't had a stroke or heart attack.

She spent four days in the hospital. She waited patiently for tests. She underwent an **MRI scan** of the brain and a CT angiogram with injection of IV contrast material (an x-ray-based picture of large blood vessels sometimes used to help rule out major strokes). A neurologist did an examination and informed her that he'd reviewed her MRI. She hadn't had a stroke. "It's probably your ears," he said. He left without further explanation. She was sent home with instructions to see her primary care doctor.

One might reasonably ask, Is BPPV what Ellen's doctor meant when he said "vertigo"? Despite the perception that doctors are precise, it is not always the case. In fact, vertigo isn't a diagnosis. It's a symptom. It's what you tell the doctor: "I'm spinning." This might seem on the surface to be a trivial semantic distinction. But the bigger problem is when patients are labeled as having "vertigo" with almost no further thought about what is the cause. This can lead to real problems.

Ellen's story illustrates a major challenge to our medical system. Science can help us understand disease mechanisms and even find cures, but unless the information is disseminated and practiced by the medical community, few will benefit from a scientific discovery. Most doctors have heard of BPPV, but in our experience most are not clear on exactly what it is or how to treat it. We have talked with ER doctors about BPPV, and many indicate that their job is to identify and treat life-threatening illnesses, not "benign" disorders. Certainly, most patients with BPPV don't think their condition is benign.

If you go to an ER anywhere in the United States with typical symptoms of BPPV, you are ten times more likely to undergo a CT scan of the brain than to receive the simple positioning test to identify BPPV (this test is described below). How does this happen? What can we do about it? Obviously, one solution is better education of doctors and patients. But information about BPPV is widely disseminated in medical texts and all over the Internet. There are more than 40 videos posted on YouTube demonstrating the treatment maneuver. Changing a medical system that rewards diagnostic tests and procedures much more than it rewards talking to patients and performing simple bedside physical examination is another important solution.

What Can I Do to Help My Doctor Make the Diagnosis?

One question you may have is whether you will remember your symptoms when it comes time to see a doctor. This may be a problem because, while the core symptoms are fairly simple to describe, they may be harder to observe when you have nausea and the world is spinning violently. Do not despair if you cannot precisely recall your symptoms when you first think about it. BPPV can be distressing. Over time you will learn the small details. You will be better able to describe these details to your doctor.

Once a diagnosis of BPPV is suspected, it is easy for a trained doctor or vestibular physical therapist to confirm the diagnosis by doing an examination. The **Dix-Hallpike test** is now familiar to most doctors. In this test, the person sits and turns the head about 45 degrees to one side. The person then lies down on his or her back, so the head ends up bent off the edge of the bed or table. The test is repeated on the other side. The affected side is the side that triggers the typical vertigo. In some cases, both sides trigger vertigo, suggesting that there is debris in the semicircular canals of both ears, which does, rarely, occur! The physical signs of BPPV mirror the symptoms. After a brief delay lasting only seconds, there is a flurry of rhythmic jerking eye movements called **nystagmus**. To the trained eye, this nystagmus makes the diagnosis. There is no other medical problem that causes this exact type of eye movement. We suggest you try to record or have someone record your eye movements after position change (when you are having the vertigo) with a smartphone camera, and show the recording to the doctor. Such a recording can potentially save a lot of time and effort.

The signs of BPPV can be intermittent. A single negative examination for BPPV does not rule it out. If a person describes recent symptoms (within the past week, say) that strongly suggest BPPV, we sometimes have him lie down for several minutes and then repeat the test. The rest period allows the debris to coalesce into a clump. Or we may have the person come back for a follow-up test on a different day. Also important to note is that the condition can spontaneously resolve without treatment, though of course our preference is to treat it, as it can persist for many months in some people.

Most people with BPPV have the calcium-containing debris (many people say "crystals") trapped in the back canal (the posterior semicircular canal) of the inner ear. But if you are unlucky, you may be one of the minority with debris in your horizontal semicircular canals. Horizontal canal BPPV may feel a little different from the more common posterior canal variant of BPPV. After a position change, the wave of dizziness may last several times longer (a minute or more) than it does with the more common posterior canal variety of BPPV. The spinning can be severe and often is associated with nausea. The treatment for horizontal canal BPPV differs from the treatment for posterior canal BPPV. The test for horizontal canal BPPV is simple. You lie on your back and turn your head to the side, first with the right and then left ear down. If someone looks at your eyes, they will see jerking eye movements (nystagmus) beating either toward or away from the ground (toward one side of your head, rather than toward the top of your head as occurs with the previously described and more common posterior canal BPPV) when you turn to the right and left. The abnormal side is the side with the most severe vertigo and nystagmus. Again, you can take a video to show your doctor. You probably will need to see a trained professional for treatment of the horizontal canal variant of BPPV, but you can try sleeping on the normal side (the side that produced the least vertigo) for several nights. In many cases this allows the debris to fall out of the affected horizontal canal.

What Laboratory Tests Should My Doctor Order and Why?

This answer is easy: usually, none. As noted above, the diagnosis is made at the bedside with the Dix-Hallpike positional test. Typically there is no need for special goggles or a video eye movement recording system such as **videonystag-mography** (VNG). Your doctor should in most cases easily see the nystagmus with the naked eye. Rarely, BPPV can be associated with other inner ear diseases, in which case it might be appropriate for your doctor to order a hearing test and an inner ear balance test (for example, VNG or rotational test) to see if there is damage unrelated to the loose otoconia that are causing BPPV. If your examination uncovers red flags (see below), the doctor might consider an MRI of the brain.

What Is the Best Treatment for BPPV?

The only proven effective treatment for BPPV (involving the posterior semicircular canal) is the Epley maneuver, and other similar **canalith repositioning maneuvers** designed to roll the debris out of the semicircular canal back into the utricle. Before doing an Epley maneuver, you first need to know which ear is affected. In most cases where BPPV affects only one ear the person has vertigo and nystagmus upon moving from the sitting position to the head-hanging position with the affected ear down toward the ground. The modified Epley maneuver shown in figure 2 is essentially an extension of the Dix-Hallpike test. After the vertigo subsides in the affected-ear-down position, the person rolls across toward the unaffected ear, ending up with the nose facing the ground. During the roll the head must be kept down as much as possible, preferably below the level of the table or bed. This second position is held for about 30 seconds and the person then returns to the sitting position. Vertigo can occur in any of the three positions (affected ear down, nose down, or return to sitting), but it tends to be most pronounced in the initial affected-ear-down position. The maneuver is repeated until there is no vertigo or nystagmus in any position.

Other treatment maneuvers such as the Semont maneuver also work, but there have not been as many controlled treatment trials as with the Epley maneuver. Some doctors still recommend the Brandt-Daroff exercises, in which the person with BPPV sits on the edge of a bed and repeatedly lies down on the right and left sides. Brandt-Daroff exercises are easy to describe and easy to perform, but unfortunately they are not effective. The canalith repositioning maneuvers are not exercises but rather a specific treatment for BPPV and are only performed when the person is having positional vertigo. Once the vertigo subsides, the maneuvers are stopped (often after a single maneuver). Meclizine can provide symptomatic relief and may be taken before the Epley maneuver to decrease nausea and vomiting during the maneuver, but it does nothing to the underlying mechanical problem in the inner ear. Multiple types of maneuvers have been used to treat the less common horizontal canal variant of BPPV with varying success, but the simplest is to sleep on the normal side (the side with less nystagmus and vertigo) for a few nights. If symptoms persist, you will need to see a specialist in dizziness treatment.

What Can I Do on My Own to Treat BPPV?

Can BPPV be treated at home without the help of a health care provider? This is a difficult question. The answer is probably yes, assuming it is the typical variety without any unusual features. Can you do any harm if you do the Epley maneuver incorrectly or you don't have BPPV? Probably not, but this does bring up an important point. The maneuver only works for BPPV, not for other causes of vertigo. The first step is to have a correct diagnosis. In our experience, the paper handouts given to patients by their doctors in an effort to treat BPPV are often not very helpful. It is difficult to understand the drawings or to get the head positioned just right while the world is spinning around violently.

Once a person with BPPV has been seen and treated in our clinics, we often give instructions on how to perform a treatment maneuver at home should they have a recurrence of BPPV (see figure 2). We also may instruct people who have had BPPV always to avoid positioning their head in any position where the head is extremely far back (below flat), to decrease the possibility that debris will fall back into a semicircular canal. You may want to avoid situations such as having your hair washed in a bowl at the hair salon or hanging upside down for any reason. In general, though, we try not to restrict people's activities too much, as many of the exercises that might lead to BPPV have other benefits (e.g., yoga and other floor exercises).

There is no need to sleep propped up after performing maneuvers to treat BPPV. You can do anything, including flying in an airplane, as long as you avoid hanging your head below a flat surface. As noted above, there are multiple videos on the web illustrating the BPPV treatment maneuver, including the ones from the American Academy of Neurology, which are well done. The bottom line, though, is this: if BPPV proves difficult to treat, a person will benefit from seeing a professional versed in treating BPPV, either a doctor or a vestibular physical therapist.

When BPPV is severe, people are sometimes unable or afraid to get out of bed. The slightest movements in bed may cause violent vertigo, making it all but impossible to get up. Once one does get up, a different kind of dizziness (usually a sensation similar to motion sickness) may take over and linger throughout the day. This often improves over several hours, only to return when the victim goes back to bed in the evening. All too frequently, we get a message from a patient with BPPV,

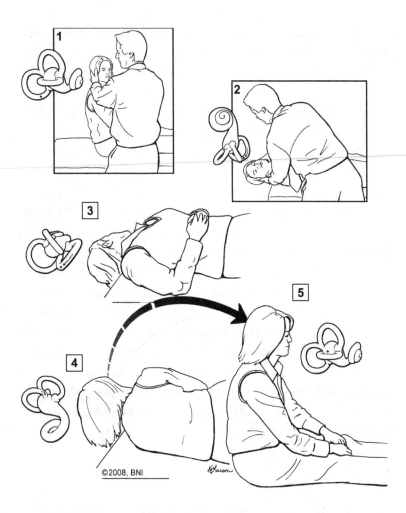

Figure 2 Modified Epley maneuver for treating right-sided BPPV. For left-sided BPPV, begin with the head turned to the left and, after falling back to the left, roll from left to right. Used with permission from Barrow Neurological Institute, Phoenix, AZ

saying something like, "I was cured 6 months ago, but it's back." We say, "Come in. We'll fix it." The patient says, "That's impossible. I can't get out of bed." What to do? If you have ever had BPPV, we recommend having a bottle of meclizine available. You don't need a prescription for meclizine. It's available over the counter. Ask a pharmacist. You may never need it. But if you are ever faced with the prospect of being unable to get out of bed because of a recurrence of BPPV, at least you can take the edge off the symptoms enough to be seen by a doctor or possibly to do the maneuver on your own.

Talk with your doctor about getting through the treatment. Some people find it difficult to get through the repositioning treatments such as the Epley maneuver, particularly if they are extremely sensitive to motion sickness or prone to panic attacks. There is an answer to this problem. Your doctor can prescribe anti-nausea or anti-anxiety medications before performing maneuvers to treat BPPV. As noted above, meclizine is available over the counter, and it can be taken at least 30 minutes before treatment to lessen symptoms. The use of meclizine does not affect your doctor's ability to accurately perform an examination for BPPV or anything else. We have found that if adequate medication is provided, anyone can get through treatment for BPPV. If you are pre-treated with medication, you may not be able to drive afterward, so bring someone with you to the appointment.

BPPV Mimics

It is unlikely for an experienced doctor to mistake BPPV for any other diagnosis. However, doctors who do not regularly treat dizzy patients may use the term in a nonspecific fashion to refer to just about any cause of vertigo. A key point is that BPPV tends to occur in bed. If you do not have brief dizzy spells triggered by getting into bed or turning over in bed, then you should question the diagnosis of BPPV. Similarly, if you have sudden vertigo spells while sitting or standing without moving your head this is probably not BPPV.

Vertigo of any cause can be aggravated by position change or by lying on one side or the other. **Vestibular migraine**, for example, often occurs on first awakening in the morning and the vertigo is usually worse when lying on one side. The key difference between vestibular migraine and BPPV is that the vertigo persists in all positions, including sitting and standing, and it is not associated with the typical position triggered nystagmus of BPPV. **Central positional vertigo** can be associated with a variety of neurological disorders that involve the middle part of the cerebellum, the balance center of the brain. The vertigo attacks can be brief like with BPPV, but unlike BPPV they occur in all head-back positions and usually there are other associated neurological symptoms. Nystagmus associated with central positional vertigo, or central positional nystagmus, is nearly always downbeating (with the fast phase of the nystagmus beating toward the feet). An experienced doctor should easily differentiate it from BPPV nystagmus. Rarely, positional vertigo can be triggered by compression of a vertebral artery (one of the arteries that run up the back of the neck to supply the back of the brain) with extension or rotation of the neck. In the rare condition called **rotational vertebral artery syndrome**, turning the head compresses a vertebral artery, leading to compromised blood flow to portions of the brain stem and/or cerebellum. As with other types of central positional vertigo, the nystagmus with the rotational vertebral artery syndrome is downbeat, and there are usually other associated neurological symptoms.

Red Flags

- Positional vertigo is equal in all head-back positions.*
- Epley maneuver has been tried on multiple occasions without any benefit.*

- Other associated symptoms such loss of vision or double vision, numbness or weakness of an arm or leg, clumsiness of the arms or legs, or slurring of speech.*
- Nystagmus is downbeating.*

*Any of these symptoms suggests a possible central nervous system cause for the positional vertigo.

CHAPTER 2

Orthostatic Hypotension

While standing, you suddenly feel lightheaded, like you might faint. The symptoms improve when you sit or lie down (just the opposite of BPPV). The dizziness may be more noticeable first thing in the morning or after standing for long periods of time, particularly on a hot day. Symptoms may be related to taking medications that lower heart rate or blood pressure.

For thousands of years, doctors commonly performed bloodletting as a therapeutic intervention. This intervention likely contributed to or caused the deaths of millions of people. George Washington was bled four liters within ten hours before his death for treatment of a throat infection in 1799. As in many other areas of medicine, the story of how bloodletting began to fall out of favor apparently began at least partially in Europe. The nineteenth-century French doctor Pierre Piorry devised rules about which patients should be bled and which should not. In 1830, it was common to perform bloodletting even in patients with blood loss from trauma. Piorry recognized that this practice only made the problem worse. In his writings, he described coming upon a man who was unconscious after bleeding from a traumatic injury. Well-meaning relatives had propped him up to make him more comfortable.

Piorry laid the man flat, and he immediately, almost magically, woke up. With his "lying down therapy," Piorry recognized that gravity could help or hinder blood circulation to the brain.

Several decades after Piorry's discoveries, the idea that low blood flow to the whole brain could cause medical symptoms was beginning to get some attention on the other side of the Atlantic. In 1917, while chair of the Harvard University department of physiology, Walter Cannon published a brief note in the journal *Science* observing that the release of adrenaline by the adrenal glands increases heart rate and blood pressure. Cannon coined the term "fight-or-flight response" to describe the situation in which a threatened animal experiences a cascade of automatic responses (including the release of adrenaline) that increase the chance of escape and survival. A key part of the fight-or-flight response is the ability to maintain sufficient blood flow to brain.

As far as the average American doctor was concerned, however, it was unclear whether these changes in the autonomic nervous system were an important cause of medical symptoms or just a curiosity of the physiology laboratory. That was about to change. As the 1920s roared in, a few American doctors reported phenomena similar to those Piorry had noted years earlier in France. In the first issue of the *American Heart Journal*, published in 1925, Samuel Bradbury and Cary Eggleston, working at the Cornell Division of Bellevue Hospital in New York, described three patients whose blood pressure—and therefore, presumably, blood flow to the brain—dropped to dangerously low levels when standing, causing the patients to have fainting episodes. During subsequent decades, doctors called this condition Bradbury-Eggleston syndrome. In modern parlance, we would say these patients had a failure of their automatic neurological reflexes, also known as dysautonomia, leading to **orthostatic hypotension**. Orthostatic hypotension means that upon moving from a lying down to either a sitting up or standing position, there is a substantial and sustained decrease of blood pressure.

Orthostatic hypotension symptoms result from abnormally low blood flow to the brain. It's easy for the heart to pump blood downhill to the legs, abdomen, and pelvis, but pumping blood uphill to the brain when you are on your feet takes more work. As you might imagine, depriving the whole brain of blood can cause a broad range of symptoms, including dizziness and weakness. People with orthostatic hypotension describe their dizziness as a lightheaded, woozy, or near fainting sensation. The affected person may feel hot, and there can be associated sweating and nausea; in extreme instances, the person may actually faint. Almost everyone has jumped up from a lying or sitting position and felt a brief lightheaded sensation. This is more likely to occur on a hot day or after lying in bed for a long time. A variety of cardiovascular reflexes typically kick in automatically to increase blood pressure and heart rate so that the lightheaded sensation is brief.

What factors might predispose a person to develop orthostatic hypotension? The most common factor is dehydration, which technically means a deficiency of water. A more accurate term for what commonly happens is intravascular volume depletion—not enough blood in your blood vessels to supply your whole body, including your brain. In other words, your tank is low. There are many causes of dehydration, from not drinking enough water on a hot day to chronic illnesses or medications that decrease intravascular volume. Blood may pool in the legs, abdomen, and pelvis, particularly with lack of exercise. With anemia there may be adequate blood volume but not enough oxygen being carried in the blood going to the brain. Any prescription medication that lowers blood pressure (intentionally or not) can predispose a person to orthostatic hypotension. We find that the more blood-pressure-lowering medications a person is on, and the higher the doses of these medications, the more likely that person is to develop orthostatic hypotension.

Although dehydration and blood pressure medications are the most common causes of orthostatic hypotension, there are many other less-frequent causes. Sometimes, the parts of the nervous system that regulate blood pressure and blood flow are damaged. These blood-flow-regulating structures and their associated reflexes are part of the autonomic (or automatic) nervous system—the system that regulates heart rate, blood pressure, blood flow, and other internal body processes (e.g., sweating, digestion, and respiration)—so we are free to ignore them. Imagine if you had to deliberately change your heart rate and blood pressure on standing. The autonomic nervous system ensures that these vital functions occur effortlessly. The autonomic nervous system acts like a team of traffic cops, directing blood flow here, there, and everywhere to ensure you have enough blood in the muscles to run when needed, enough blood in the digestive system to process your food after a meal, and enough blood going to your brain, which is always working hard. A wide range of medical conditions can damage the autonomic nervous system and cause orthostatic hypotension. Some of these conditions begin in or preferentially involve the nervous system, and some do not. The list of conditions associated with orthostatic hypotension includes **Parkinson disease**, peripheral neuropathy (disease of the peripheral nerves, e.g., nerves of the arms and legs), and inherited neurological disorders that involve the autonomic nervous system. People with these conditions may have severe orthostatic hypotension and may not be able to stand for more than a few minutes without blacking out. Sometimes people only notice problems when they have to stand for a long period of time, such as waiting in a line.

It is well known that astronauts who spend time in weak gravity—called microgravity—such as on the International Space Station, develop orthostatic hypotension on returning to Earth. Humans evolved with gravity. We respond adaptively to the constant pull of gravity acting on us. On Earth, when you stand up, about half a liter of blood moves from your chest to your legs, abdomen, and pelvis and up to a quarter of your blood volume moves out of blood vessels into the tissues, decreasing blood return to the heart. In response, pressure sensors in the blood vessels and gravity sensors in the inner ear and abdomen signal the autonomic nervous system to activate corrective reflexes that increase vascular tone (i.e., pressure exerted by the muscles surrounding blood vessels) and heart rate, which delivers more blood flow to the brain. Astronauts' autonomic nervous systems must change their settings for cardiovascular reflexes in space and again when they return to Earth. This can take several hours to several days. A similar phenomenon explains why people develop orthostatic hypotension following prolonged bed rest and why it can take several days to readjust to standing up.

Why is orthostatic hypotension more common in older people? One answer is that older people are more likely to be taking medications that interfere with cardiovascular reflexes and lower blood pressure. As a general rule, for people receiving antihypertensive medications, the diastolic—the "bottom number" in the blood pressure reading—should not be below 70 and never below 60. The decision on what is the best blood pressure for you can lead to disagreements between your cardiologist and neurologist. In most cases, the heart loves low blood pressure, the lower the better, but the brain needs adequate pressure to maintain blood flow, particularly when standing. Complicating matters further, older people often have narrowing of the small arteries deep in the brain so that even higher pressure than is generally considered ideal may be needed to get blood through these narrowed arteries. A trial of lowering the dose of or discontinuing blood pressure–lowering medications should always be considered in older people with orthostatic hypotension. Inactivity and lack of exercise is another common contributor to orthostatic hypotension in older people. A regular exercise program can prevent pooling of blood in the lower extremities and improve blood return to the heart even in older people with varicose veins. Finally, older people are much more likely to develop neurological disorders that predispose to orthostatic hypotension including Parkinson disease and related disorders, and peripheral neuropathy.

Typical Symptoms of Orthostatic Hypotension

Dizziness with orthostatic hypotension is typically described as lightheadedness, swimming, wooziness, faintness, or a feeling of an impending faint. This is sometimes associated with feelings of generalized weakness and shakiness. When severe, orthostatic hypotension symptoms may include blurring, tunneling, or darkening of vision; headaches; irritability; anxiety; and generalized weakness. As mentioned above, many forms of dizziness are induced or aggravated by moving from a lying down to a sitting position. However, when a person complains of lightheadedness on moving from a sitting to a standing position, it is a strong possibility that the person has orthostatic hypotension or other disorder of autonomic nervous system function. A key feature of orthostatic hypotension is that the symptoms are alleviated by sitting or lying down and by squatting.

A more serious symptom of orthostatic hypotension is a faint or **syncope**. Syncope may be defined as a sudden, brief loss of consciousness due to a drop in blood flow to the whole brain, usually leading to collapse followed by prompt recovery. Patients may simply report that they felt lightheaded and the next thing they knew they were on the ground. Did they lose consciousness? This can be a difficult question to answer unless there was a witness who can describe the event. Often the best we can do in these situations is to ascertain what a person felt immediately before and immediately after an episode of syncope. We like to ask the question, "What is the last thing you remember?" The sensation of an impending or near faint is called presyncope.

In most cases, if you faint, you will end up on the ground. This is usually a good thing. If you're on the ground, the heart can more easily pump blood to the head. Put simply, it's your brain's strategy to protect it from decreased blood flow. The main concern with fainting is that you might hit your head during the fall, resulting in injuries such as bone fractures or concussion. If a person faints but remains upright, such as in a telephone booth, or if well-meaning bystanders attempt to keep the person upright, the person could experience a seizure or brain damage because of a prolonged period of decreased blood flow to the brain. If a person faints, the best thing a bystander can do is to place the fainter into a flat position with feet propped up, with no attempt to prop up the head. When the person is fully awake, it may be appropriate to offer sips of water, if the person can drink safely without choking, which is always a concern in semiconscious people.

Up to half of all people will faint or have near-fainting episodes at some time in their lives. As noted earlier, nearly everyone has experienced a brief near faint sensation when jumping up rapidly from a sitting or lying position. More than

1 percent of emergency room visits are for syncope. Although orthostatic hypotension is a common cause of syncope and near syncope, there are many other potential causes, including a wide range of cardiac and neurological disorders, that emergency room doctors must consider.

CASE EXAMPLE: It's Not Always That Simple

> William is 75 years old and a retired police officer. He has known his doctor for 30 years. Over the years, they have worked to get his blood pressure under control, ultimately settling on a combination of three different medications. Now, when William comes in for a physical examination, his blood pressure is "normal," usually around 130/60. However, William has increasingly felt weak. He can't pinpoint any particular part of his body that is weak—maybe his legs—but really he just feels weak all over. At times he feels lightheaded, particularly just after getting up or after being on his feet for more than a half hour. He doesn't feel as mentally sharp as he used to. His doctor suggested at one point that he might have orthostatic hypotension, but he checked orthostatic vital signs (blood pressure and pulse lying down and standing up) in the office, and everything was "fine." William has undergone a 12-lead EKG (a common heart test, performed by attaching electrodes to the chest and monitoring the electrical impulses of the heart), a 24-hour EKG called a Holter monitor, and a heart stress test. Everything was normal. He is a "medical mystery."

We hear this kind of story frequently in our dizziness clinics. It can be a diagnostic dilemma. In our experience, many such people do better with three simple interventions: sufficient consumption of water, regular exercise, and less medication. The latter can be a tough sell. We all know that keeping blood pressure low prevents many undesired outcomes: heart attack, stroke, and hemorrhages. Yet, as noted above, there is such a thing as too low blood pressure, particularly in older people. That William needed multiple blood pressure medications in the past does not mean he still requires those medications.

A simple trick is to spend a few extra minutes taking the vital signs. What works well is to have a person lie down for a few minutes and measure blood pressure and heart rate. Then, the person should stand in one place, as though the feet are glued to the floor, for at least three minutes while blood pressure and heart rate are measured at least once per minute. During this period of observation, the person should be asked whether any symptoms are being experienced such as dizziness or a subtle blurring of vision that wasn't there while lying down. Another common sign of orthostatic hypotension is excessive swaying when a person stands in one place for too long. This swaying—really a form of imbalance—may be behind the documented positive association between orthostatic hypotension and risk of falls in older people. In one study, older people for whom the systolic blood pressure (the top number) fell by at least 20 mm Hg within one minute of moving from a lying-down to a standing-up position had a significantly higher risk of falling within one year, compared to those who did not experience such a drop in blood pressure on standing up.

To "push the envelope" with this test, the person can be asked to try to stand for longer periods of time, which often reveals more subtle versions of orthostatic hypotension. A drop in blood pressure that occurs after more than three minutes of standing is sometimes called delayed orthostatic hypotension. Delayed orthostatic hypotension may be a milder form that often progresses over time to orthostatic hypotension that occurs more within three minutes (the ordinary definition of orthostatic hypotension somewhat arbitrarily requires that the drop in blood pressure occurs within three minutes of standing). Sometimes it is also helpful in the diagnosis of a person who feels dizzy while standing to ask her to lie down or squat, to see if the symptoms go away. Caution: having a person stand up from a squatting position can provoke a faint. It is best to do this under medical supervision to ensure safety.

What Can I Do to Help My Doctor Make the Right Diagnosis?

The diagnosis of orthostatic hypotension is made when the systolic blood pressure—the "top number" in the blood pressure reading—drops more than 20 mm Hg or the diastolic blood pressure—the "bottom number" in the blood pressure reading—drops more than 10 mm Hg within three minutes after you stand up from a lying-down position. Ordinarily to make this diagnosis, a doctor would want to see the decrease in blood pressure persist for at least a couple minutes, or at least not rely too much on any single blood pressure reading. If the drop in blood pressure is accompanied by typical symptoms of orthostatic hypotension that were not present when you were lying down, confidence in the diagnosis is increased. You can help your doctor by taking your blood pressure and pulse on your own at home when you are having symptoms. Automatic devices for recording blood pressure and pulse are readily available in drug stores at reasonably low cost. We recommend using the ones that go around the arm rather than those that go around the wrist. Often, the most prominent abnormalities occur in the early morning. You can take blood pressure and heart rate readings first thing in the morning, while lying in bed, and then after standing up next to the bed. It is also helpful to measure blood pressure and heart rate at times when symptoms are most severe and to compare these to values obtained when symptoms are least severe.

One of the key facts that your doctor must know when considering the diagnosis of orthostatic hypotension is whether you are taking medications that might make it likelier that you will develop orthostatic hypotension. It is therefore imperative for you to create and maintain an up-to-date list of your medications and take it with you to the doctor visit. Include on your list the doses of medications and when each medication was started and when doses were changed. As noted above, medication adjustments may have a major beneficial impact on orthostatic hypotension.

What Laboratory Tests Should My Doctor Order and Why?

As with BPPV, the answer, usually, is none. The diagnosis is made at the bedside by taking blood pressure and pulse measurements in the lying-down and sitting-up positions and again after you have been on your feet for several minutes. Sometimes it can be helpful to perform an EKG at the same time, if there is a question of a slow or irregular pulse rate. A tilt-table test is another possibility; in this test the patient is strapped securely on a table that can tilt from a horizontal (lying-down) position to a near vertical (standing) position, such as 60 degrees up from horizontal, while blood pressure, pulse rate, and EKG are continuously monitored. This type of testing can be useful if the patient's symptoms are atypical or if bedside testing is equivocal. However, some normal people may develop near faint dizziness or even faint on a tilt table. If a person faints or nearly faints on a tilt table, the technologist is trained to return the person to a lying-down position to facilitate a quick recovery.

What Is the Best Treatment for Orthostatic Hypotension?

Unless you have a medical contraindication (a reason not to, such as congestive heart failure), your doctor may advise you to add extra water and/or sodium (salt) to your diet. For many people, consumption of at least 1.5 liters of water per day (at least six eight-ounce glasses) is appropriate as a treatment for orthostatic hypotension. Addition of sodium is a little trickier. Although the effects of adding sodium are similar to those of consuming water, there is a greater tendency for increased sodium to raise blood pressure. When adding sodium, it should be determined whether the person with orthostatic hypotension has high blood pressure while lying down (so-called supine hypertension). With supine hypertension and orthostatic hypotension, you are between a rock and a hard place. The goal is to raise blood pressure while standing, but blood pressure is already too high when lying down. For people with normal supine blood pressure, doctors often start by prescribing approximately 1 gram of sodium three times a day, but like any other treatment, this would need to be adjusted to suit the individual person's needs. This extra sodium consumption can often be accomplished by eating foods with salt; salt tablets are usually unnecessary.

If you do have supine hypertension, how can this be addressed? Raising the head of the bed by placing the bed frame safely and securely on solid objects may help. It provides some tilt training for you at night, which may induce your system to respond better to being upright in the day. It also decreases the blood pressure in the brain relative to the lower extremities and pelvis due to gravity. You should discuss this approach with your doctor. Another approach is to take a low dose of short-acting blood-pressure-lowering medication before going to bed so its effects will be going away by the next morning when you get up. At a minimum, it will be important for your doctor to document what you are doing and when you are doing it. This type of information can be invaluable later in adjusting treatment.

If orthostatic hypotension symptoms persist despite conservative treatment such as increasing water and salt intake, your doctor may prescribe a medication to increase blood pressure. The most commonly prescribed drugs are fludrocortisone and midodrine. Fludrocortisone works by increasing blood volume, while midodrine works by increasing vascular tone—that is, contraction of the smooth muscles in the walls of the blood vessels. With severe orthostatic hypotension, a combination of the drugs may be used since they have different mechanisms of action. In addition there is a longer list of less commonly used medications that may be appropriate in select individuals.

Because some of the medications used in treatment of orthostatic hypotension run the risk of inducing or aggravating supine hypertension, your blood pressure should be checked frequently when these medications are started. One approach is to check blood pressure after lying down for at least an hour, as well as first thing in the morning lying down, first thing in the morning standing up, and midday while standing up, to gauge the likely range of blood pressures.

One expects to see the highest blood pressures lying down and the lowest blood pressures on first standing up in the morning; a goal of treatment should be to moderate the extremes of blood pressure. Your doctors may want to look at a series of blood pressures taken either in the clinic or office or at home. A series of blood pressure measurements on different days is always more useful than a single measurement. The medications described above are typically given during the day, when higher blood pressure is beneficial, and avoided at night, when there is a risk of dangerously high blood pressure while lying down. If you are taking fludrocortisone, you may need blood tests of potassium and magnesium, which should be monitored by your doctor, so stay on top of your blood tests the best you can. Keep all your results in a folder or notebook. If you are due for a blood test and nobody has called you, take the initiative to call and ask somebody about it.

What Can I Do on My Own to Treat Orthostatic Hypotension?

The simplest things you can do to treat orthostatic hypotension are maintain good hydration and exercise regularly. Drink plenty of water when exercising on a hot day. Regular exercise improves muscle tone and prevents blood pooling in the lower extremities and pelvis. Thigh-high compression stockings and abdominal compression garments can also improve blood return, though they can be a challenge to put on and uncomfortable to wear, particularly on a hot day.

Orthostatic hypotension is often most severe first thing in the morning. You should sit on the edge of the bed for a minute or so, then get up slowly. It may help to have a glass of water at the bedside and drink it before getting up. If you experience symptoms while standing and cannot easily sit or lie down, you can try "counter maneuvers," such as crossing your legs, raising up on your toes, tensing your thighs and buttocks, or bending forward. Other times at which people may be at an increased risk for orthostatic hypotension include immediately after meals, after exercise, and after getting upright from a bent-forward or squatting position. Excessive heat should be avoided, especially first thing in the morning. Some people with orthostatic hypotension may benefit from changing the time of a warm shower from early morning to later in the day.

Orthostatic Hypotension Mimics

Cardiogenic syncope, syncope caused by heart disease, is the greatest fear when a doctor sees a patient who faints or has a near faint spell. When we were in training, we admitted almost all first-time syncope patients to the hospital overnight because of concern about a serious heart problem. These patients almost never had anything serious going on but instead had experienced a common faint. However, it's still a good idea to be cautious and do some investigation, at least with the first episode of fainting. Heart problems essentially can be divided into those of electricity and those of plumbing. Electrical problems involve the heart's electrical activity, "the wiring." These may cause a sudden increase or decrease of heart rate, either of which affects the heart's pumping ability. Another type of electrical problem is disease of the electrically active heart muscle, which can be due to multiple causes, such as coronary artery disease or previous viral infection of the heart muscle. Heart plumbing problems can be divided into those that interfere with blood supply to the heart itself and those that interfere with blood supply to everywhere else, including the brain.

With **vasovagal syncope** (also known as neurocardiogenic or neurally mediated syncope) the heart may inappropriately slow down so much that it can't pump enough blood to the brain (cardioinhibitory phenomenon). This condition produces the most symptoms when the peripheral blood vessels also inappropriately dilate so that not enough blood returns to the heart (vasodepressor phenomenon). As a result the blood flow to the brain drops so low that the person faints. Some people unwittingly precipitate vasovagal syncope by abruptly arising from a seated position at just the wrong moment. For example, a person having dinner with friends in a restaurant may feel lightheaded and then become anxious and jump up from her seat in an effort to get away from the social situation and avoid embarrassment, thereby unintentionally triggering vasovagal syncope. Excitement such as seeing a nurse coming toward you with a large hypodermic needle is another common trigger for vasovagal syncope. Curiously, episodes of vasovagal syncope often cluster. They may occur multiple times in one month and then disappear as mysteriously as they came.

A common orthostatic hypotension mimic that occurs in younger people is the **postural orthostatic tachycardia syndrome (POTS)**. Most people with POTS, in our practice, are under age 40, with onset of symptoms typically occurring between 13 and 19 years of age. Like with orthostatic hypotension, patients with POTS develop a range of symptoms when standing, including lightheadedness and near faint dizziness, all relieved by sitting or lying down. Other associated symptoms include headache, mental clouding ("brain fog"), heart palpitations, blurred or tunnel vision, tremulousness, and severe fatigue. Unlike with orthostatic hypotension, patients with POTS do not have a drop in blood pressure with standing (it may even increase) but rather a marked increase in pulse rate. The diagnosis rests on finding a sustained increase in pulse rate of more than 30 beats per minute (more than 40 beats per minute, by some criteria) within ten minutes after standing, without a significant drop in blood pressure. A unique feature of POTS not usually seen with orthostatic hypotension is acrocyanosis, a dark red-blue discoloration of the legs most notable below the knees (and sometimes arms) that occurs in approximately half of patients with POTS.

As with orthostatic hypotension there are many pre-disposing factors for POTS, including blood volume loss, de-hydration, prolonged bed rest, and medications that impair the autonomic nervous system. Often, however, no cause can be identified. POTS is a syndrome not a disease, and there are clearly multiple mechanisms for causing symptoms. Some pa-tients with POTS have chronic low circulating blood volume, while others have chronic elevated levels of norepinephrine consistent with a hyperadrenergic state. The term "hyperad-renergic" indicates excesses of epinephrine and norepineph-rine, which lead to excessively high heart rates.

As with orthostatic hypotension, the first line of treat-ment for POTS is consumption of adequate quantities of non-caffeine-containing fluids, plus exercise. Because patients with POTS are usually younger and in most cases do not have heart disease, fluids and salt can often be increased with little risk. A regular exercise program is probably the single most effective long-term treatment for POTS. Compression stock-ings (ideally up to and including the abdomen) can also help prevent pooling of blood and enhance venous return to the heart and presumably support blood flow to the brain. Cur-rently, there are no FDA approved drugs for directly treating POTS, but fludrocortisone and midodrine have been reported to be effective in some cases. Low doses of the beta blocker propranolol can be effective in lowering standing pulse rate, but higher doses are counterproductive.

Finally, as noted above, neurological conditions can dam-age the autonomic nervous system and lead to orthostatic hypotension. A variant of Parkinson disease called **multiple system atrophy** can begin with severe orthostatic hypoten-sion before other symptoms develop. Most patients with typical Parkinson disease have orthostatic hypotension to some degree, but it is rarely the predominant symptom. A wide range of peripheral neuropathies (diseases of the nerves) can involve the autonomic nervous system, including **diabetic neuropathy** and **autoimmune neuropathies**. These disorders are usually associated with other symptoms, including numbness, burning, and weakness, but one variant of autoimmune neuropathy selectively involves the autonomic nervous system, and in that case orthostatic hypotension may be the predominant symptom.

Red Flags

- Evidence of congestive heart failure: swelling of ankles, shortness of breath, chest discomfort.*
- Known cardiac valve disease.*
- Known cardiac arrhythmia (any abnormality of the rhythm of the heart, of which there are many).*
- Diagnosis of Parkinson-like syndrome.**
- Other symptoms of autonomic nervous system dysfunction: severe constipation, abnormal sweating, urinary frequency and urgency.**

*Any of these symptoms can result in decreased blood flow to the brain and mimic orthostatic hypotension.

**Orthostatic hypotension is likely due to a more widespread nervous system disorder.

PART II DIZZY SPELLS THAT OCCUR IN ATTACKS BUT WITH NO APPARENT TRIGGER

CHAPTER 3

Ménière's Disease

You have severe episodes of vertigo lasting three to four hours. These episodes come on without any apparent cause, and they continue no matter what you do. The attacks are typically accompanied by nausea and vomiting and by decreased hearing, fullness, and tinnitus (a roaring sound) in one ear. Over time the hearing in that ear becomes progressively worse.

Prosper Ménière was a French doctor who while working at a deaf mute institute in Paris was struck by the observation that vertigo and hearing loss often occurred together. In his initial report before the Imperial Academy of Medicine in 1861, he described a young man who had violent attacks of vertigo, nausea, and vomiting, without any apparent cause. Later the young man noticed loud noises in the ears, along with decreased hearing. "I could not forget that beyond the middle ear there exists an apparatus [the inner ear] which, mysterious as it is, has not revealed to us all the phenomena which takes place in it," Ménière noted.

Did the young man described by Ménière have what has become known as Ménière's disease? The modern diagnostic criteria for Ménière's disease include attacks of vertigo with one-sided ear fullness, roaring tinnitus, and hearing loss typically lasting hours. The key to the diagnosis is to document a decrease in hearing in the involved ear during an attack and a gradual progressive hearing loss between attacks. Ménière's subject had vertigo attacks followed by tinnitus and fluctuating hearing loss, but apparently his hearing loss involved both ears. The hearing loss with Ménière's disease typically begins in one ear and remains so for many years; only a small percentage of patients develop involvement of both ears, and then only after many years, typically. It is possible that the young man had some other inner ear disorder, such as autoimmune inner ear disease, but Ménière provided too few details about the case to allow modern diagnosticians to be sure.

Ménière also described autopsy findings on a young girl who suddenly developed one-sided deafness and vertigo and died five days later. The brain and spinal cord were normal, but he noted blood filling the semicircular canals of the inner ear on the side of the deafness. In retrospect this was likely a case of acute leukemia with bleeding into the inner ear, but based on Ménière's report, the concept that Ménière's disease was caused by hemorrhage into the inner ear persisted well into the twentieth century. Ménière wasn't suggesting that this young girl with sudden deafness and vertigo had the same disease as the young man with episodic vertigo, tinnitus, and fluctuating hearing loss. He was simply making the point that vertigo and hearing loss commonly occur together with inner ear disease.

In the United States of the nineteenth century, there was little or no appreciation that the inner ear played a role in balance. For example, in 1890, Howard Ayers gave a lecture at the Marine Biological Laboratory at Woods Hole, Massachusetts, titled "The Ear of Man: Its Past, Present, and Future." He discussed the anatomy of the inner ear, including the semicircular canals and otolith organs, which we now know to be the anatomical sites where physical motion is sensed and transformed into signals passed on to the brain. Ayers thought these organs were important for hearing but not balance. "The function of audition [hearing] certainly belongs to the ear; not so, however the equilibrious [balance] function . . . there is no longer the slightest evidence in favor of the theory [of the inner ear as a balance organ]."

One problem that plagued Ménière and the other doctors who wanted to study the inner ear during autopsies in the middle of the nineteenth century was the denseness of the bone that surrounds the inner ear. They could not make thin cuts through the tissue of the inner ear as was typically done to study other organs of the body with a microscope. Ménière sawed through the bone surrounding the inner ear and grossly examined its structure. The blood was easily seen but not the fine structure of the inner ear. The German otolaryngologist Karl Wittmaack solved this problem and revolutionized the study of the inner ear diseases in the early 1920s. During an autopsy he removed a cylinder of bone containing the inner ear and slowly decalcified the bone with 1% nitric acid over several months. Once x-ray analysis showed the bone was completely decalcified, he embedded the tissue in cellulose and then made thin serial cuts. Doctors from all around the world visited his laboratory to learn the technique, including a young otolaryngologist from England, Charles Hallpike (the same Hallpike that the Dix-Hallpike test, described in chapter 1, is named after).

In December 1934, a 63-year-old dockworker was referred to the department of neurosurgery at the Royal London Hospital to have his vestibular nerve cut in an attempt to stop his debilitating attacks of vertigo caused by Ménière's disease.

Along with the vertigo, he had tinnitus and progressive hearing loss in the left ear. At that time it was common to group all inner ear causes of vertigo under the label of Ménière's disease. Whether there was a Ménière's disease with specific pathology or whether there were many diseases that caused the same combination of symptoms was unknown. Regardless, in this case it was reasonably clear that the symptoms were originating from the left ear, and other people with Ménière's disease had been successfully cured of vertigo by cutting the vestibular nerve.

The operation was performed by Dr. Hugh Cairns, one of the few neurosurgeons in the world able to perform such a delicate procedure. Cairns was an Australian who attended medical school at Adelaide University and trained with the famous American neurosurgeon Harvey Cushing at Peter Bent Brigham Hospital in Boston on a Rockefeller Traveling Fellowship. (Cairns, who served in the Australian Army Medical Corps in World War I, later commented that Gallipoli and the Battle of the Marne were nothing compared to the physical stress of his neurosurgical residency with Cushing.) Cairns operated on the dockworker on December 18, 1934. He noted that the opening was smaller than usual because of the thickness and hardness of the bone, but he was able to cut the left vestibular nerve. The patient had unusually high blood pressure during the operation; that evening he became restless and then unresponsive. Despite heroic efforts to relieve pressure in the brain with a second operation, he died three days later. An autopsy performed six hours after death showed massive bleeding into the brain. Cairns cut out the inner ears in their bony capsule with a saw and placed them in storage in formaldehyde solution.

The bone pieces containing the inner ears of the dockworker sat in formaldehyde for more than a year before Cairns became aware of Hallpike's interest in inner ear pathology. After carefully scrutinizing Hallpike in a lengthy interview, Cairns decided to entrust him with the specimens. The decalcification process took about six months, and then finally Hallpike was able to cut the specimens and examine the tissue under a microscope. He observed a prominent distention of the entire inner ear sac, a condition called **hydrops**.

Just as Hallpike was preparing his exciting findings for publication, Cairns provided him with a second set of bone specimens from a similar patient who died of complications after surgery. This patient also had hydrops of the inner ear sac. The fluid within the inner ear (**endolymph**) is constantly being formed and resorbed to maintain a normal balance in pressure. Hallpike and Cairns speculated that either too much fluid was being made or there was abnormal absorption leading to increased pressure and hydrops. The increased pressure in the inner ear could explain the sense of fullness and the progressive hearing loss, but the mechanism for the sudden spells was unexplained.

Hallpike and Cairns published what they thought was the first description of the pathology in Ménière's disease in October 1939. Unknown to them, however, a Japanese otolaryngologist named Kyoshiro Yamakawa had reported similar findings of hydrops in a patient with Ménière's disease who died of pneumonia. Yamakawa, who also had studied with Wittmaack in Germany, initially presented the findings at a medical congress in Kyoto, Japan, in April 1938, publishing them in a short article in German later in the year. That investigators in Japan and England were unaware of each other's work seems inexplicable in our modern computerized age. However, in the late 1930s not only were communications slow, but there was an almost complete interruption of international exchanges in the lead-up to World War II.

So by the 1940s there was general consensus on the clinical features and the pathology of Ménière's disease, but little was known about the mechanism for producing hydrops and how hydrops caused attacks. Subsequent autopsy studies in patients with Ménière's disease have reliably found hydrops, though occasionally hydrops has been found in patients without typical symptoms of Ménière's disease. Based on the assumption that increased fluid pressure in the inner ear causes Ménière's disease, clinicians have tried many ways to lower inner ear pressure (see below).

What is the difference between Ménière's disease and hydrops (also called endolymphatic hydrops)? Some doctors will tell patients that they have hydrops instead of Ménière's disease. Ménière's disease is defined by symptoms and physical signs on examination. (Signs are what a physician can observe and test for, such as the patient's inability to detect a very low pitched sound; symptoms are what a patient experiences, like an attack of vertigo.) By contrast, hydrops is a term used to describe the pathology of the inner ear as seen at autopsy under a microscope. We prefer to use the term "Ménière's disease" when providing people with a diagnosis, reserving the term "hydrops" for autopsy findings. As MRI scans improve, and we are better able to see enlarged fluid-filled spaces in the inner ear, in the future it may also be possible to tell people whether or not they have hydrops.

Some have suggested that Ménière's disease can involve just the hearing or balance parts of the inner ear, so-called cochlear or vestibular Ménière's disease. Yet despite the large number of cases that have now been studied at autopsy, none has shown hydrops restricted to just the cochlea or just the vestibular part of the inner ear. Hydrops involves the entire inner ear. Most likely, Ménière's disease includes a wide range of signs and symptoms, with some people experiencing more hearing loss than vertigo, others experiencing more vertigo than hearing loss, and still others having an equal mixture. It's pretty clear that Ménière's disease is highly variable, affecting different parts of the inner ear in ways that vary from individual to individual, although this observation remains to be formally evaluated in research studies. As an aside, many of the people who had been diagnosed with vestibular Ménière's disease (without any hearing loss) actually have a migraine variant that has been called migraine-associated dizziness or, more recently, vestibular migraine (discussed in chapter 4).

Ménière himself first suggested a possible relationship between migraine and Ménière's disease, noting that many of his patients with vertigo and hearing loss also had migraine. Subsequently, multiple reports have indicated that migraine is more common in people with Ménière's disease than in the general population. The nature of this relationship is poorly understood, however. Does migraine lead to hydrops, or does it simply mimic Ménière's symptoms? Migraine may just be one of several risk factors for developing Ménière's disease.

Typical Symptoms of Ménière's Disease

Ménière's disease is a syndrome, defined by a combination of symptoms and findings. Attacks often begin with a sensation of fullness and pressure accompanying decreased hearing and roaring tinnitus in one ear. Vertigo rapidly follows, reaching maximum intensity within minutes but then gradually resolving, typically over a period of hours. In the early stages, the one-sided hearing loss is reversible between attacks, but over time the hearing loss continues between attacks. The tinnitus that is often compared to the sound of the ocean or a seashell next to the ear can be constant, but it often becomes louder with an attack. Nausea and vomiting typically accompany the vertigo, and balance is impaired. As we have seen, however, variations in this typical pattern of symptoms are not uncommon. Isolated attacks of vertigo or hearing loss can precede the characteristic combination of symptoms for months or (rarely) years. With one variant, called delayed Ménière's disease, vertigo episodes develop many years after the person has experienced a sudden one-sided deafness.

CASE EXAMPLE: When Is the Right Time to Consider Surgery?

> Linda is 35-year-old accountant who has experienced attacks of vertigo for the past three months. They have become incapacitating. In each case, she missed work for two or three days. She can't go on like this. She has noted hearing loss in her left ear along with roaring tinnitus that comes and goes. She knows she is about to have an attack because her left ear feels full and the tinnitus becomes louder. Then the room starts spinning, and within a few minutes she has severe nausea with repeated vomiting. She has to lie in bed perfectly still and wait for the symptoms to lessen. She was given meclizine to take at the onset of one attack. It helped a little, but she still could not function during the attack. She saw an otolaryngologist about a month ago, and he concluded that she had Ménière's disease. He gave her a prescription for a diuretic, but she has had three attacks while on the medication. She was told there is nothing more that can be done besides surgery. She is scheduled to have her vestibular nerve cut next month.

Sometimes we facetiously say that one of our roles as neurologists in a field dominated by surgeons is to save patients from surgery. The actual situation is that the authors of this book work closely with surgeons—mainly otolaryngologists (including those who subspecialize in the ear—otologists—and neurotologists). There is a constant flow of patients back and forth between our clinics and theirs. Both our specialties have something to offer people with dizziness. We often have extended discussions about the right time for surgery, particularly in patients with Ménière's disease. One reason is that spontaneous remissions are common in Ménière's disease, even if medical treatments are not effective. We typically recommend at least three to six months of medical treatment before considering invasive treatments, including surgery. However, each person with Ménière's has to be judged independently. The pros and cons of different medical and surgical treatments are discussed below.

What Can I Do to Help My Doctor Make the Diagnosis of Ménière's Disease?

The most important thing you can do to help your doctor is to carefully note the details of your attacks of vertigo. How long do the episodes last? In what circumstances do they occur? Are they associated with ear symptoms such as change in tinnitus, change in hearing, or ear fullness? With these symptoms do you also experience headache or excessive sensitivity to light and sound (i.e., photophonophobia)? If you have had prior testing, particularly a hearing test, make sure you have a copy to give to the doctor. As with other causes of vertigo attacks, it can be helpful with diagnosis to make a video recording of your eyes during an attack using a smartphone.

What Laboratory Tests Should My Doctor Order and Why?

By a long shot, the most important test is an audiogram (a hearing test performed in a sound proof room). The diagnosis of Ménière's disease rests on finding a characteristic hearing loss in the low frequencies. Other audiometric tests such as electrocochleography (ECog) and otoacoustic emissions may be abnormal, but there are too many false positives and false negatives for them to be reliable as an audiogram as an indicator of Ménière's disease. Vestibular tests such as video-nystagmogram (VNG) and electronystagmogram (ENG) can identify damage to the vestibular part of the inner ear and are sometimes helpful when invasive options like injections or surgery are being considered (since the patient and physician want to know how much vestibular function remains and whether the damage is just on one side).

What is the role of MRI in diagnosing Ménière's disease? At present, its main duty is to rule out other causes of a one-sided hearing loss such as a benign tumor of the vestibular nerve called an acoustic neuroma or **vestibular schwannoma**. These benign tumors rarely cause much vertigo but instead typically present with a gradually progressive one-sided hearing loss. A good rule is that most people with a newly recognized major asymmetry of hearing should be considered for an MRI. When an MRI is done to rule out an acoustic neuroma, it must be done with contrast (colloquially also known as a dye injection) because these small tumors can be missed without contrast enhancement. Current MRIs do not visualize the tiny inner ear well enough to see hydrops, but new techniques with a special detector coil near the ear are being developed to improve resolution of the images of the ear that can be obtained by MRI. Preliminary studies at UCLA have shown that improvement of hydrops on MRI correlates with improvement in clinical symptoms. MRI could revolutionize both the diagnosis and treatment of Ménière's disease. It would provide a "gold standard" to evaluate and compare different treatments.

What Is the Best Treatment for Ménière's Disease?

The first line of treatment for Ménière's disease is a medication to suppress symptoms at the time of an attack. Symptomatic treatments such as meclizine, dimenhydrinate, and diazepam do not prevent attacks, but they do seem to reduce the severity and duration of symptoms in a Ménière's-related attack. These medications should be taken at the earliest sign of onset of an attack, before severe nausea and vomiting occur. Once vomiting occurs, medications can be given via suppositories or injection since oral medications will not be absorbed.

Salt-restriction diets and **diuretics** were the earliest treatments and continue to be the most prescribed treatments for preventing Ménière's attacks. Clearly, some patients with Ménière's disease are exquisitely salt sensitive, but this is a subset. Prolonged salt restriction in all people with Ménière's disease is of questionable benefit. However, a trial of salt restriction should be the first line of treatment. The effectiveness of diuretics has never been proven in adequately controlled treatment trials, but most clinicians feel these medications are effective at least in some patients. We typically prescribe either triamterene with hydrochlorothiazide or acetazolamide and recommend a three-to-six-month course before deciding on efficacy. Migraine is common in patients with Ménière's disease, and acetazolamide has the added benefit of treating both migraine and Ménière's disease.

In his frustration with current medical treatments for Ménière's disease, a colleague recently noted that everything cures Ménière's disease and nothing cures Ménière's disease. He was referring to the fact that the natural course of Ménière's disease is so variable and spontaneous remissions are so common that it is difficult to know if a medication is effective or improvement is by chance alone. That's why there are so many claims for "miracle" cures for Ménière's disease on the Internet—yet not one of them has stood the test of time and been proven effective in controlled treatment trials. We are not nihilistic regarding treatment of Ménière's disease. We simply urge you to be cautious in accepting claims of cures based on testimonials. As the saying goes, if it sounds too good to be true, it probably is.

Based on the finding of hydrops in patients with Ménière's disease, surgeons have tried a wide range of procedures to drain fluid from the inner ear (such as endolymphatic shunt surgery). These procedures have largely been abandoned because of the technical difficulty of maintaining a functioning drainage tube in such a small fluid compartment (about 1 cc of fluid). Assuming there is an inflammatory component to Ménière's disease, doctors have injected steroids into the middle ear through the eardrum, where the medication can make its way into the inner ear. A controlled treatment trial is currently under way to see if this treatment works, but it will be a while before we know the results. Cutting the vestibular nerve (i.e., vestibular nerve section) is a reliable way to stop the vertigo attacks with Ménière's disease, since the abnormal signals set off by the hydrops cannot be passed on to the brain. Surgical techniques have improved since the time of Cushing and Cairns, so major complications are rare, but this is still brain surgery and should not be taken lightly.

Of course, vestibular nerve section does not treat hydrops. The intent of the surgery is to selectively cut the vestibular nerve and avoid damage to the cochlear nerve carrying hearing information from the ear to the brain. The hearing loss and ear noises will continue even though vertigo stops. Most patients will compensate for the loss of vestibular function on one side, but it can take months for the brain to "rewire" so that balance returns to normal. Rare patients compensate poorly after surgery and become chronically dizzy. A less invasive way to obtain the same result is to inject gentamicin through the eardrum into the middle ear where it slowly crosses into the inner ear. This procedure is called intratympanic gentamicin injection. Gentamicin is an antibiotic that is selectively toxic to the vestibular part of the inner ear. For some years now, this has been a popular procedure in Europe, where studies found that about half of patients will obtain good results with a single injection. The popularity of intratympanic gentamicin injection is growing rapidly in the United States. It has all but replaced surgery in some practices. People may require multiple injections to control vertigo, and some are not helped, presumably because the drug does not make its way into the inner ear. It is important to point out that only a small minority of people with Ménière's disease will require injection or surgery. Most obtain acceptable relief of symptoms with a combination of diet and diuretics.

What Can I Do on My Own to Treat Ménière's Disease?

The cornerstone of initial Ménière's disease treatment is careful management of sodium (or table salt) intake. Study the label of every food you buy for sodium content. Processed foods are often very high in sodium content, so use fresh foods as much as possible. Aim for about 500 mg of sodium per meal and no more than 2,000 mg of sodium per day. It is a good strategy to spread out consumption of sodium over the course of each day. Don't load all your sodium consumption into one meal such as dinner. People with Ménière's tend to do well with smooth, regular consumption of sodium rather than sudden intake of large amounts of sodium. It also may be a good strategy to ingest fluids over the course of the day. Avoid binge drinking of fluids. A slow, steady consumption of water throughout the day may help prevent dizziness. If you are doing vigorous cardio exercise, you may find you do better sipping on water throughout your workout—or, if you sweat a lot, you may want to use an electrolyte-containing drink. The goal should be to keep your fluid and sodium levels nearly constant at all times. Some people with Ménière's disease will improve greatly with these dietary modifications. For those who do not, your doctor may prescribe a diuretic.

You should have a contingency plan for what to do if you unfortunately do get an attack of vertigo. You should have one or more medications on hand that suppress vertigo and nausea. This may be as simple as over-the-counter meclizine. Or your doctor may prescribe other medications to be used alone or in combination. You should have a plan to get help when you need it. Make sure you have access to people, which usually means a cell phone. It goes without saying that if you have an attack, you will want to rest, try to breathe in a relaxed fashion, and adjust the temperature of your environment to whatever is most comfortable to you. If you are unable to keep fluids down for a prolonged period of time, you may need IV fluids, but this rarely happens.

Ménière's Disease Mimics

Any disorder that causes a combination of vertigo and hearing loss could mimic Ménière's disease. **Autoimmune inner ear disease** can start with vertigo attacks and fluctuating hearing loss, but the course of symptoms is much more aggressive than with typical Ménière's disease, with progressive severe hearing loss on both sides within the first few months. Typically the hearing loss will respond dramatically to steroids or other immune suppression. Autoimmune inner ear disease can be part of a systemic autoimmune disorder such as lupus or rheumatoid arthritis, or it can selectively involve the inner ear. As noted above, **migraine** can mimic Ménière's disease; in a very small subset of people it may even cause Ménière's disease. Chronic infections of the inner ear, including latent syphilis, can also mimic Ménière's disease, but as with autoimmune inner ear disease, the course is much more aggressive than with typical Ménière's disease.

Red Flags

- Slowly progressive hearing loss without fluctuations; difficulty understanding speech. These symptoms might be caused by a vestibular schwannoma, a small benign tumor on the eighth cranial nerve.
- Hearing loss in both ears early in the course. These symptoms could be caused by a more aggressive disorder such as autoimmune inner ear disease or chronic infection.
- Associated neurological symptoms (e.g., loss of vision, slurred speech, weakness of face, arm, and/or leg on one side). These could be symptoms of a **transient ischemic attack (TIA)**.

CHAPTER 4

Migraine-associated Dizziness

Over the past three years you have had approximately ten spells of vertigo, nausea, and vomiting. On those days you spent most of your time in bed. By the next day the vertigo was gone. You have been very susceptible to motion sickness since childhood, and you have experienced migraine headaches since your early teens. You are sensitive to light and sound with some of the vertigo spells, but you don't have headaches.

The observation that migraine and dizziness often occur together dates back to the nineteenth century when Edward Liveing noted their connection in his classic book *On Megrim, Sick-headache, and Some Allied Disorders*. Liveing studied mathematics and medicine at Cambridge and developed his "nerve storm" theory of megrim (migraine) in the mid nineteenth century. In a nutshell, he felt that migraine was similar to other paroxysmal neurological conditions such as epileptic seizures, vertigo attacks, and trigeminal neuralgia—all caused by a sudden discharge within the brain, a nerve storm. Although his theory on the mechanism of migraine has largely been abandoned, he provided a detailed description of symptoms seen in patients with migraine, including dizziness and motion sickness. Only in recent years have we recognized how common dizziness is in people with migraine. Migraine-associated dizziness affects at least 1 percent of the general population, and about two-thirds of people with migraine headaches have a lifelong sensitivity to motion sickness.

Dizziness can occur during headaches, but it often occurs during headache-free intervals. Only about one-quarter of patients usually experience headaches with their dizziness. Migraine-associated dizziness attacks typically last from hours to days, but there can be a baseline dizziness that never completely goes away. If the person with migraine-associated dizziness is seen by a doctor during an attack, the doctor may note nystagmus with similarities to that of a person who has either an inner ear problem or a brain problem. We really don't understand why patients with migraine are so prone to dizziness, nor do we understand the basic cellular mechanisms of migraine, with the notable exception of a few rare families with documented genetic mutations.

Migraine headaches and migraine-associated dizziness share many common features. Both are much more common in women. Attacks of both migraine headaches and dizziness can be precipitated by changes in barometric pressure, lack of sleep, fasting, certain foods, and emotional stress. Many with migraine-associated dizziness have relatives with migraine headaches and dizziness. Moreover, medications that are effective for preventing migraine headaches are often effective in preventing migraine-associated dizziness.

When we first suggest to a patient that their dizziness may be related to migraine, they typically are skeptical. "But I haven't had a migraine headache for several years," they maintain, or "I don't get headaches with my dizzy spells." Our response is that migraine is not a headache. It's a disease, a genetic disease. The most common symptom is headache, but not everyone with migraine gets headaches. Some may have episodes of flickering lights in their visual field, called a visual aura. Headaches may follow, but sometimes the visual aura is the only recognizable symptom of migraine, often called ocular migraine. We frequently see people who tell us, "I don't have migraine headaches, I have ocular migraine." The reality is that if you have any of these migraine symptoms, you have the genetic disease called migraine, and the challenge is to find ways to live with and manage the symptoms.

Similar to ocular migraine, recurrent, spontaneous bouts of vertigo, nausea, or motion sickness may be a migraine-equivalent symptom that can occur with or without headache. Genetic mutations that cause migraine have been identified in families with a rare variant of migraine, called hemiplegic migraine. People in these families have spells of numbness and weakness on one side of the body associated with headaches. Others in the same family have just migraine headaches with or without visual aura. The genetic variants that cause more common types of migraine have yet to be identified, but there clearly are multiple genes—some that increase susceptibility and others that decrease susceptibility to developing migraine symptoms. The pattern of genes in the family determines which symptoms individuals will have—visual aura, vertigo attacks, or just extreme sensitivity to motion sickness.

Multiple environmental factors can trigger migraine symptoms in genetically susceptible individuals. Female hormones are particularly important triggers for migraine symptoms. This explains why migraine symptoms tend to be more prominent in women. Headaches are usually most frequent and severe during menstruating years and improve after menopause. Other common triggers include barometric pressure change, temperature change, stress, lack of sleep, excessive exposure to heat, and going a long time without eating. It is important to separate triggers from cause. Stress will not cause migraine symptoms in someone who does not have the genetic susceptibility to develop migraine.

Typical Symptoms of Migraine

Almost everyone has a friend or family member with migraine headaches. The affected person prefers to take to bed in a quiet, dark room, often with a cold wet cloth over her eyes. People experiencing migraine prefer to lie perfectly still because motion triggers nausea and even vomiting. A person with migraine may have multiple types of headache. The headaches with nausea and sensitivity to light described above are only the tip of the iceberg. In our neurology clinics, so-called chronic sinus headaches are nearly always due to migraine. It is worth noting that a sizable number of patients with migraine in the United States have probably undergone questionable sinus surgery based on a misdiagnosis of sinus disease. Only about one-third of people with migraine are aware that they have migraine. The definition of migraine involves having had, over your lifetime, at least five headaches that were bad enough to cause you to stop your normal activities and that were associated with either nausea (sick headache) or excessive light and sound sensitivity (photophonophobia). Obviously, there are other causes for bad headaches (see list of red flags at the end of this chapter), particularly a first bad headache, but if you have had headaches with these features over several years and nothing else has developed, you have migraine.

Migraine headaches can be preceded by a visual aura and, as noted above, sometimes the visual aura occurs without headache. There are many types of visual aura, but two of the most common are a scintillating scotoma, which is a blurred or blind arc in the visual field with a shimmering zigzag border (figure 3), and a fortification spectra, which is a visual hallucination with jagged edges that resemble a fortified town with bastions around it. These visual auras, which typically last 20 to 30 minutes, are more specific for the diagnosis of migraine than the headaches.

Migraine is associated with a wide range of dizziness symptoms. The most common by far is sensitivity to motion, both self and surround motion. Motion sensitivity typically begins in childhood with episodes of car sickness and persists throughout life, sometimes with sudden worsening later in life. Some people with migraine cannot ride in an automobile unless they are driving and find it difficult to work on a computer because motion on the screen triggers dizziness and nausea. Most people with migraine have symptoms of motion sickness during their headaches, and some will have spontaneous episodes of motion sickness without headache or any apparent trigger.

Dizziness attacks with migraine take several forms, from a spinning sensation to a nonspecific dizziness and imbalance. Nausea and vomiting are common with all varieties of migraine-associated dizziness. The typical duration is hours to days, but episodes can be brief, and people may report sudden sensations of a tilt in the surroundings so that they feel as though they may fall. Dizziness attacks can be associated with headache or light and sound sensitivity but can occur without any other migraine symptoms. Ear fullness, tinnitus, and in some cases even ear pain are common in people with migraine; while these symptoms might suggest an ear disease, hearing is usually not affected by migraine (unlike in Ménière's disease, where a one-sided hearing loss is required for the diagnosis).

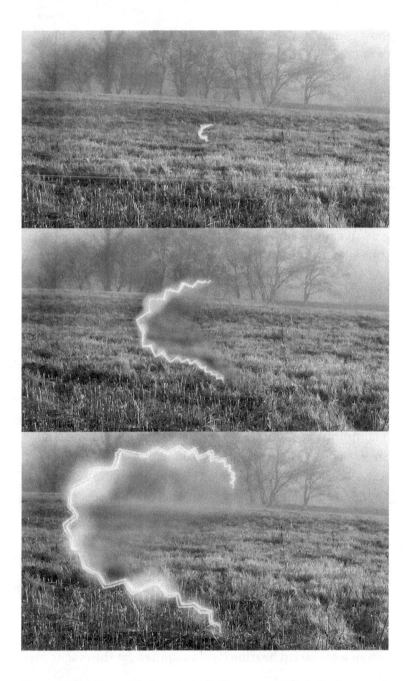

Figure 3 Migrainous visual aura (scintillating scotoma). Typically the area of visual distortion gradually enlarges over 10 to 30 minutes and then spontaneously resolves.

Grace, a 38-year-old teacher, has experienced recurrent dizzy spells that date back as far as childhood. Her most recent spell occurred on a rainy day at school, and she had to lie down in the nurse's office for a few hours before her husband was able to come and take her home. She took a meclizine tablet that she always carried with her. This took the edge off of the vertigo, nausea, and vomiting, but she still could not carry on her normal activities and was eventually able to fall asleep at home. The next morning she was back to normal. She has had up to four of these spells a year for the past 15 years, and she noticed that she was more likely to have a spell if there was a change in barometric pressure, if she was stressed, or if she did not get adequate sleep. Usually the spells would subside if she was able to fall asleep. During the spells she was very sensitive to sounds and preferred to rest in a quiet room.

When Grace was a child she had shorter, more abrupt spells of vertigo, with projectile vomiting. These spells stopped in her early teens. Complicating matters even more, after a few of her adult spontaneous vertigo spells, she continued to have brief episodes of vertigo triggered by position change for several weeks. During one of these periods of positional vertigo, a doctor examined her and identified the typical positional nystagmus of BPPV. The positional vertigo she'd experienced stopped after the doctor performed an Epley maneuver.

Grace also had a prior history of migraine headaches that started when she began menstruating and now occurred less frequently and never with her vertigo attacks. There was a family history of migraine headaches in her mother, maternal grandmother, and two siblings. A maternal aunt and one of her siblings had vertigo spells, and the aunt was told she had Ménière's disease.

Grace experienced three different types of vertigo attacks and also had a personal and family history of migraine headaches.

Why do we think the vertigo spells have anything to do with migraine? After all, migraine is common. Maybe the vertigo attacks are caused by some other inner ear problem unrelated to migraine. These are valid questions. Let us examine each of a few vertigo types separately.

The syndrome of benign recurrent vertigo of childhood was first described in the early 1960s. A young child, often under the age of four, suddenly becomes frightened, cries out, clings to the parent or staggers as though drunk, sweats profusely, and vomits. Most have difficulty describing what they are experiencing, but some report spinning. The attacks typically last minutes and then the child returns to playing as though nothing had happened. The possibility that this might be a migraine-equivalent syndrome was suggested in the initial report, but it wasn't until years later that follow-up reports documented that nearly all of these children developed typical migraine symptoms. Furthermore, no other cause was ever found. Other migraine-equivalent syndromes in children include recurrent bouts of abdominal pain, cyclical vomiting (without vertigo), and episodic double vision.

As with vertigo in children, benign recurrent vertigo in adults has been linked to migraine primarily by association— nearly all cases have a personal and family history of migraine—and typically no other cause can be found. Furthermore, as noted above, the vertigo attacks have many features in common with migraine headaches, including associated light and sound sensitivity, triggers such as stress and lack of sleep, and response to migraine preventative medications. How migraine causes vertigo attacks or headaches is poorly understood. We are just beginning to identify the genetic factors that make a person more likely to develop migraine, and the common thread is an increased excitability of nerve cells in the brain. Consistent with this observation is the observation that people with migraine tend to be hypersensitive to all sensory stimuli including light, sound, smell, and motion.

Finally, what does migraine have to do with BPPV? As noted in chapter 1, BPPV is a mechanical abnormality of the inner ear—dislodged otoliths enter a semicircular canal and move with position change. BPPV is common in older people, but when it occurs in younger people it is strongly associated with migraine. Several studies have found that more than 50 percent of people with BPPV under the age of 50 have migraine. Between 10 and 15 percent of the general population have migraine. Since BPPV is clearly a disorder of the inner ear, somehow migraine must damage the inner ear. One possible explanation is reversible spasm of the arteries supplying the inner ears, causing transient decreased blood flow. So-called vasospasm is known to affect arteries to the brain and eyes in some people with migraine, causing transient neurological symptoms or transient blindness in one eye. Of note, vasospasm of the brain arteries that supply the ear might be expected to cause both spontaneous episodes of vertigo and later development of BPPV, as transient decreased blood flow to the inner ear is known to release otoliths from the otolith organs.

What Can I Do to Help My Doctor Make the Diagnosis of Migraine-associated Dizziness?

As with other causes of dizziness, probably the most important thing that you can do to ensure a correct diagnosis is to be observant during an attack. How did it begin? How long did it last? What did you feel? Were there other symptoms? Keep a log describing each attack at the time it occurs. Also note whether you have had other migraine symptoms, particularly headaches, light and sound sensitivity, or visual aura and motion sensitivity, either with the dizziness attacks or separately. Use your smartphone or another device to make a brief video recording of your eyes during the spell.

What Laboratory Tests Should My Doctor Order and Why?

The diagnosis of migraine-associated dizziness rests on identifying the characteristic symptoms described above and ruling out other likely causes. There is no specific test for migraine-associated dizziness. Probably the most important related condition to rule out is Ménière's disease, which by definition requires a particular type of one-sided—or at least asymmetric—hearing loss. An audiogram (hearing test) should be obtained. Imaging of the brain is not required unless there are red flags suggesting other neurological disorders.

What Is the Best Treatment for Migraine-associated Dizziness?

Most people with migraine-associated dizziness will benefit from a symptomatic medication such as meclizine or dimenhydrinate to be taken at the onset of attacks. Promethazine suppositories are useful for people with severe nausea and vomiting who cannot absorb oral medications. These drugs "take the edge off of symptoms" but do not stop an attack. They should not be taken daily, since they do not prevent attacks. Triptans (such as sumatriptan and rizatriptan) that abort migraine headaches have not been adequately tested for migraine-associated dizziness. Investigators at UCLA are currently conducting a placebo-controlled treatment trial to see if rizatriptan will abort migraine dizziness spells.

Your doctor might consider a trial of a migraine preventative drug, although these drugs have only been tested in controlled studies for headache; there have only been anecdotal reports of benefit for migraine-associated dizziness. Several classes of drugs including antidepressants, anticonvulsants, beta blockers, and calcium channel blockers have been shown to cut down the frequency and severity of migraine headaches. These drugs take several weeks to become maximally effective. Only by taking them consistently for at least that long can a person reliably decide whether the medication is successful or not.

What Can I Do on My Own to Treat Migraine-associated Dizziness?

The first line of treatment of migraine-associated dizziness is to manage triggers as much as possible. A regular exercise program helps with stress and improves sleep. Stress-management techniques such as meditation and yoga can also be helpful. Long periods without eating can trigger migraine symptoms, so be sure to eat something for breakfast and lunch. A range of foods and food additives can trigger migraine symptoms in select individuals; migraine diets have been developed. It is common sense to avoid anything that triggers symptoms, although extreme dietary restrictions are rarely helpful. We do recommend that people experiencing migraine associated symptoms avoid binging on caffeine. Caffeine withdrawal is a known trigger for migraine symptoms, so if you use caffeine it should be used in moderation and on a regular basis. Those who feel that living with minimal caffeine is impossible can look for inspiration to Tom Brady, the well-known American football player, who in 2016 surprised fans by announcing that he has never had a cup of coffee.

Mimics of Migraine-associated Dizziness

As noted above, migraine-associated dizziness is partly a diagnosis by exclusion, meaning that the physician must be sure there are no other likely causes for the dizziness attacks. **Ménière's disease** can have identical vertigo spells but also has those unilateral (one-sided) ear symptoms, including fullness, roaring tinnitus, and hearing loss. Patients with migraine-associated dizziness commonly have fullness and ringing, but in *both* ears, and hearing remains normal. Vertigo spells can occur with many neurological disorders, including **multiple sclerosis, transient ischemic attacks (TIAs)**, and **brain tumors**, but invariably there are other associated neurological symptoms, and the symptoms progress with time (for stroke and TIAs, see chapter 6).

Red Flags
- One-sided hearing loss could be Ménière's disease or some other inner ear disorder.
- Sudden change in headache pattern could be another neurological disorder.
- Associated neurological symptoms could be a stroke or TIA.
- First-ever severe headache, with or without loss of consciousness, could be a ruptured brain aneurysm.

PART III   A SINGLE BOUT OF DIZZINESS THAT LASTS FOR DAYS THEN GRADUALLY IMPROVES

CHAPTER 5

Vestibular Neuritis

You notice a gradual buildup in vertigo over several minutes. You then develop generalized sweating and severe nausea followed by vomiting. You try to walk to the bathroom but have to hold on to objects to keep from falling. These symptoms are severe and continuous for about three days and then begin to improve gradually. Even after a few weeks, you still feel slightly unsteady when walking, and you notice brief dizziness if you turn your head quickly to one side.

In a classic paper published simultaneously in England and the United States in 1952, Dix and Hallpike described the typical symptoms associated with what they called vestibular neuronitis. Hallpike was an otolaryngologist in London who along with Cairns first described the inner ear pathology associated with Ménière's disease. Margaret Dix was a young researcher working with Hallpike at the Queen Square Neurological Institute in London. She had been in surgical training but was disfigured in the bombing of London during World War II and decided to focus on a career in research. Unlike Ménière's disease, which involved recurrent attacks of vertigo, vestibular neuronitis was characterized by a single prolonged bout of vertigo lasting several days to weeks. Dix and Hallpike chose the term "vestibular neuronitis" because they felt that the damage causing the vertigo was probably localized to the vestibular system, the nerve cells or nerve fibers outside or inside the brain. Their conclusion was based on the observation that patients with vestibular neuronitis had isolated vertigo without hearing or neurological symptoms. The ending "-itis" in medical jargon suggests inflammation, and usually infection—thus implying an inflammation or infection of the vestibular system. Yet Dix and Hallpike admitted that they had little or no information about the cause of the disorder.

As in the case of Ménière's disease, the key information regarding the cause of vestibular neuronitis came from studies of inner ear specimens obtained at autopsy from patients who had typical symptoms of vestibular neuronitis and later died of other, unrelated causes. The person who was most responsible for defining the pathology of vestibular neuronitis was Harold Schuknecht, the long-time chief of otolaryngology at the Massachusetts Eye and Ear Infirmary at Harvard Medical School. In many ways, Schuknecht was the prototypical American success story. From his small-farm South Dakota beginnings where the only book in the house was a bible, he attended college and the first two years of medical school at the University of South Dakota and then transferred to Rush Medical School in Chicago to complete his training while working multiple part-time jobs to support his education. In World War II he was a flight surgeon with the Fifteenth Air Force Division in Italy, where he received the Soldier's Medal for rescuing a pilot from a burning plane. After the war Schuknecht did his residency training in otolaryngology at the University of Chicago and then stayed on to develop his clinical and research skills as an assistant professor.

After a stay at Henry Ford Hospital in Detroit, Harold Schuknecht moved to Harvard to chair the Department of Otolaryngology in 1961. He immediately set up a temporal bone (the bone at the base of the skull that contains the inner ear) laboratory and began collecting specimens at autopsy from patients with a wide range of inner ear conditions. His "Sunday school" temporal bone sessions with the resident doctors were a tradition at the Eye and Ear Infirmary. Harold Schuknecht was a workaholic. He worked long days during the week and shorter days on the weekend. He read manuscripts and wrote research papers mostly at home. He slept five or six hours a night but often woke up in the middle of the night and began writing. Schuknecht did not consider himself intellectually gifted, but he was proud of what he called his "intellectual stamina." He worked harder and stuck with things longer than others.

Schuknecht's greatest academic achievement was his textbook titled *Pathology of the Ear*, which is still considered the definitive work on what can go wrong in the ear. In it he relied on specimens from his "temporal bone bank" to describe the pathology associated with all of the common disorders of the inner ear. His discovery of the loose otolith debris in patients with BPPV was instrumental in the later development of the simple cure described in chapter 1. He had several specimens from patients with typical symptoms of vestibular neuronitis. He preferred the term **"vestibular neuritis,"** however, as he thought the disorder resulted from a viral inflammation of the vestibular nerve. There was shrinkage of the vestibular nerve fibers and loss of nerve cells of one ear similar to the pathological findings of known viral infections. He later introduced the term "neurolabyrinthitis" to cover the spectrum of viral inner ear syndromes. Some seemed to affect just the vestibular part of the inner ear, such as with vestibular neuritis, while others involved the entire inner ear, producing vertigo and hearing loss (often called **labyrinthitis**).

Based on what we know now, most cases of vestibular neuritis likely result from reactivation of a Herpes virus that lies dormant in the nerve cells of the vestibular nerve. The reactivated virus moves down the nerve fibers, causing swelling and compression of the nerve in its tight bony canal. An analogous condition is Bell's palsy, where people develop paralysis of one side of the face as the result of reactivation of a Herpes virus that lies dormant in the nerve cells of the facial nerve. Dormant Herpes viruses can be found in nerve cells of both the facial and vestibular nerves in many people. Why the virus becomes activated is not completely understood, but changes in the immune system likely play a role. A wide range of viruses are capable of causing labyrinthitis with combined auditory and vestibular loss. The clinical course for vertigo and imbalance is similar for vestibular neuritis and labyrinthitis. Full recovery takes weeks to months. With labyrinthitis there is the additional hearing loss on one side, which often remains permanent.

Typical Symptoms of Vestibular Neuritis

Over a period of minutes to hours a person with vestibular neuritis develops severe dizziness, typically described as a violent spinning of the environment. This dizziness is invariably accompanied by difficulty standing. The person usually requires assistance to walk but with support can stand and make a few hesitant steps. During the first 24 to 48 hours of the illness, people typically experience nausea and vomiting. They usually spend the first day in bed and are not able to eat much. Many visit an emergency room. For a few days, it may be difficult to keep food down. By the end of the first week, most people are beginning to eat solid food and take tentative steps on their own. Gradually, over a period of weeks (though everyone is different), the person continues to improve. Most but not all people are back to a normal work schedule within a few weeks. The rate of improvement varies between individuals. The kind of work the person does is important, too. Someone with a desk job might be back to work more quickly than a construction worker who has to nail shingles on a roof or operate hazardous equipment.

Vestibular neuritis is generally considered a monophasic illness, meaning that it comes on and then gradually improves without relapsing. However, patients may have a temporary increase in their dizziness, imbalance, and nausea, most notably during the first few days of their illness or to a lesser degree even months later, in the context of a severe illness such as a serious respiratory infection. Why this happens is not well understood, but we think it's because the illness undermines the brain's usual strategies to compensate for the original vestibular damage. The person nearly always returns to baseline once the new illness resolves.

About half of people with vestibular neuritis will develop BPPV (described in chapter 1) at some time during the course of recovery. BPPV presumably occurs because the viral infection causes otolith material to be dislodged and float around within the inner ear. If the debris enters your posterior semicircular canal, you develop BPPV.

CASE EXAMPLE: Pills Are Not Always the Answer

A 35-year-old busy executive with no prior illnesses was relaxing after dinner one evening when she suddenly noticed the room was beginning to spin. Over the next few hours, her balance deteriorated. She began to experience nausea, and she vomited several times. Her husband helped her to the car and drove her to the emergency department of a local hospital. In the emergency room an IV was started, and she was given fluid replacement and medication to suppress the vomiting. The emergency room doctor noticed that her eyes were moving back and forth and told her that she had nystagmus. He ordered a CT scan of the brain "to rule out stroke." When the CT scan came back normal, he told her that she probably had an infection of the inner ear and wrote a prescription for meclizine, instructing her to take it three times a day. "Don't worry," he said, "you should be back to yourself in a week or two." She was discharged home with a four-page list of standardized discharge instructions, including reasons to return to the ER. Three weeks later she was much improved, but she still felt dizzy and slightly off balance and did not feel capable of returning to work or driving. She continued to take the meclizine three times a day.

What went right and what went wrong in this patient's visit to the emergency room for typical symptoms of vestibular neuritis? A potentially serious complication of vestibular neuritis is severe dehydration from repeated vomiting, so replacing fluids and suppressing vomiting was good treatment. The ER doctor identified nystagmus and ultimately concluded that the vertigo likely originated from a benign inner ear infection, and he prescribed meclizine to suppress the severe vertigo and nausea. It is appropriate to suppress the acute symptoms with meclizine. However, this medication should only be used for the first few days, when vertigo and nausea are prominent. Long-term use of meclizine can interfere with the compensation process for the inner ear damage. People should be encouraged to return to normal activities as rapidly as possible and stop meclizine as soon as the severe symptoms subside (usually in two or four days).

Although it may sound strange, people should attempt to do activities that make them dizzy, such as rapid head turns and quick body turns. The brain needs to receive "error signals" to make the adjustments for the inner ear damage. As we discuss below, a physical therapy program with vestibular exercises can be helpful, particularly in the early recovery stage (the first few weeks). Finally, was the CT scan of the brain appropriate and necessary? The answer is probably no. The patient was a healthy 35-year-old without any known risk factors for stroke. If there were findings in the patient's history and examination to suggest the possibility of stroke then the procedure of choice would be an MRI of the brain; the types of stroke that can cause vertigo are not generally identified with a CT scan. (The brain stem and cerebellum are the areas usually involved in these types of stroke, and these areas are not well visualized with CT.) If there is any doubt, it is often useful to get a neurologist involved in the emergency room evaluation. Several major academic neurology departments are setting up "telestroke" programs that use cameras and remotely located neurologists to assist hospitals that do not have neurologists on call in the emergency room.

What Can I Do to Help My Doctor Make the Diagnosis of Vestibular Neuritis?

In the practice of neurology, timing is everything. "Intermittent dizziness for three years" means something quite different from "imbalance that has steadily worsened for three years." One of the characteristic features of vestibular neuritis is that it comes on like a slow explosion. Within hours to a few days, a normal, often highly functional person becomes incapacitated and dependent on others. This temporal pattern is often described as "maximal at onset." When dizziness and imbalance are maximal at onset and more or less improve in the days and weeks that follow, you and your doctor should at least think of vestibular neuritis as a possible diagnosis. The improvement can be slow, taking weeks and even months if the damage was severe. A person who has severe vertigo but then feels completely better the next day does not have vestibular neuritis.

Vestibular neuritis is usually defined in terms of rapid onset of persistent vertigo; indeed, the person with vestibular neuritis is usually able to describe feelings of vertigo. We say "usually" because we have seen people with vestibular neuritis in which the person reports rapid onset of imbalance rather than a sensation of spinning. There is a simple physical sign of vestibular neuritis that everyone can recognize: difficulty walking. As far as we can recall, we have never seen a convincing case of vestibular neuritis in which the person had no trouble walking in the first day or so after onset. So impaired walking is an important clue to diagnosing vestibular neuritis.

It is always a good idea to keep track of the onset and progression of dizziness symptoms, including whether there are any ear symptoms or neurological symptoms (such as confusion, loss of vision, slurred speech, weakness, numbness, tingling). If you see the doctor later in the course of vestibular neuritis, you should bring records of other doctors' notes from any ER visits or any other medical visits that occurred during the first few days of the illness. The symptoms and signs observed during the first few days often clinch the diagnosis. The physical signs decrease over time, making the diagnosis harder and harder the farther you get from the onset of symptoms. As we have noted several times, it may be possible for you to use your smartphone to take a video of your eyes to document the type of nystagmus during the early stages of the illness. That video may help your doctors with the diagnosis.

What Laboratory Tests Should My Doctor Order and Why?

When the patient is seen in the acute phase (early stages), when the patient has nystagmus and imbalance without other neurological signs, the diagnosis of vestibular neuritis can usually be made at the time of the physical examination without the need for laboratory tests. A test that your doctor can do at the bedside to confirm the diagnosis of vestibular neuritis is the head impulse test. The doctor places hands on each side of your head and then makes tiny quick movements to each side while asking you to focus straight ahead, while watching your eyes to see if they stay focused straight ahead with abrupt head movements to the right and left. With vestibular neuritis, when the head is quickly moved toward the abnormal side the eyes will move passively along with the rest of the head and your brain will have to generate a rapid corrective eye movement to bring the eyes back to straight ahead. This occurs because one of the main functions of the inner ear balance system is to keep your eyes stable when your head is moving. If there is damage to the vestibular nerve on one side, the eyes are not stable with rapid movements to that side. Unfortunately, most doctors are not experienced in performing the head impulse test and don't feel comfortable using it for the diagnosis of vestibular neuritis. An automated system with video goggles to record the eye movements and to analyze the data during the head impulse test has been developed and is being tested in emergency rooms at multiple medical centers. Preliminary studies suggest that a positive head impulse test may be more useful for ruling out a stroke than an MRI of the brain.

Videonystagmogram (VNG), which tracks eye movements using video, and electronystagmogram (ENG), which tracks eye movements using surface electrodes pasted on the skin around the eyes, are tests your doctor might consider, particularly if the physical examination tests are not definitive or if the course of your illness is atypical. VNG and ENG tests—these two tests in practical terms are the same—record nystagmus that may occur spontaneously in the dark or after stimulation of the inner ear with warm or cool water (caloric test) or with rotation of the patient on a motorized chair. A major advantage of these tests is the ability to record nystagmus with eyes open in the dark and to quantify the magnitude of the nystagmus. With acute vestibular neuritis, spontaneous nystagmus in the light with fixation disappears within a day or two, yet spontaneous nystagmus can be recorded in the dark for weeks and even months after onset. Caloric-induced nystagmus is decreased on the affected side, and rotational testing in the dark is asymmetric, with decreased response after rotation toward the affected side.

The head impulse test, rotational testing, and caloric testing are all slightly different ways of assessing the function of the vestibulo-ocular reflex (VOR). The VOR keeps images stable on your retina when your head moves. When the VOR isn't working, head movement causes vision to momentarily blur. Because of impairment of the VOR, people with vestibular neuritis often note that if they look quickly toward the side of the affected ear, their vision momentarily becomes blurred and then clears. This deficit in the VOR can be quantified with VNG or ENG.

Finally, an audiogram, or hearing test, can be helpful to be sure there is no unexpected one-sided hearing loss to go along with the one-sided vestibular loss. It is helpful to identify hearing loss if there is any and, if so, to characterize whether the hearing loss is attributable to the inner ear or to some other cause, such as a middle ear disorder.

What Is the Best Treatment for Vestibular Neuritis?

There is general agreement with regard to the effectiveness of several treatments. In the acute phase—soon after onset of symptoms—it is comforting and important to suppress the severe vertigo, nausea, and vomiting. Recurrent vomiting can lead to dehydration, which, if severe, can damage organs throughout the body. A medication called dimenhydrinate (Dramamine) suppresses both vertigo and nausea and is a good first-line treatment. It can be given intravenously (IV) or intramuscularly (IM) if vomiting is repetitive. Dimenhydrinate is more sedating than meclizine, but this is typically not a problem in the acute phase, when sedation is helpful. Medications specific for nausea and vomiting such as prochlorperazine or ondansetron can be added if vomiting is not controlled. Meclizine given orally is effective for lesser vertigo as symptoms improve in days two and three. However, as noted above, medications like dimenhydrinate and meclizine should only be used during the acute phase and should be stopped as soon as possible because they can interfere with the compensation process. As soon as acute symptoms begin to subside, vestibular rehabilitation (also known as vestibular physical therapy) should begin, ideally with the help of the physical therapist who has special training in this area. If this therapy is not available, then vestibular rehabilitation exercises appropriate for vestibular neuritis can be downloaded from the Internet.

The role of steroids and antiviral medications for treating vestibular neuritis is more controversial. A placebo-controlled clinical trial performed in Germany and published in the *New England Journal of Medicine* suggested that a course of high-dose steroids started within the first three days of onset of symptoms can improve the recovery in inner ear damage after vestibular neuritis. The problem is that there are significant risks of side effects with high-dose steroids, and it is difficult to judge the risk-to-benefit ratio for this type of treatment. Complicating matters further, patients improve symptomatically regardless of whether there is residual inner ear damage. We do not know for sure whether in the long run, steroids make any difference with regard to symptom recovery. The same study found no benefit from antiviral medications given within the first three days of onset for vestibular neuritis. As with most negative clinical trial results, it is possible that these medications would work if given at a different stage of the disease (e.g., within a few hours of onset), but we really don't know. More controlled studies are needed to address these important issues.

What Can I Do on My Own to Treat Vestibular Neuritis?

In the acute phase you need to maintain hydration by drinking fluids and suppressing vomiting. Dimenhydrinate (Dramamine) and meclizine (Bonine or Less Drowsy Dramamine) can both be obtained over the counter. As noted earlier, meclizine and related drugs are comforting during the first few days of the illness, but continuing them beyond the acute phase will almost certainly prolong the recovery process. It is critical to begin moving around as soon as possible once acute symptoms subside. In animal studies, recovery after inner ear damage on one side is accelerated if the animals are placed in a rich environment and encouraged to move about and exercise. By comparison, recovery of animals left in a dark cage without stimulation is markedly delayed. Using due caution, and with the help of friends and family, you should try to get out of bed and begin walking, more and more each day.

Similarly, the sooner you begin normal head and eye movements, the faster you will recover. A useful exercise is to stare at a target while moving your head back and forth or up and down. The speed of the head movements can be gradually increased as long as you can keep the target in focus. If you stay in bed in a dark room, your recovery will take longer. The sooner after onset of vestibular neuritis that you begin a course of physical therapy, the better you will recover in the long term, probably.

Using reasonable caution, you can begin walking on uneven surfaces like grass or sand, which is an excellent challenge for balance. Similarly, exercise programs that focus on control of core muscles are likely to be helpful. Examples of exercise programs that may help are tai chi, qigong, Pilates, and dancing, again all using caution. Many communities have balance classes, and these can be a helpful addition to vestibular physical therapy.

"When can I drive?" people recovering from vestibular neuritis commonly ask. The answer to this question requires some judgment, common sense, and respect for the unpredictability of driving situations. If you are not comfortable quickly looking around the room to see what's going on at every corner, you are probably not ready to drive. Usually a person knows when it is safe to drive, but if you have any doubt, you should not do so. Even after you decide you are safe to drive, it would be best to first try driving slowly in an empty parking lot with another driver in the passenger seat. Some communities have driver assessment programs run by an occupational therapist, and of course, your local Department of Motor Vehicles (DMV) or Registry of Motor Vehicles (RMV) is always willing to test drivers if there is any doubt.

Vestibular Neuritis Mimics

A major concern for any patient who has acute prolonged vertigo and imbalance is that he may have had a **stroke**. Obviously the likelihood of a stroke is much higher in an older person with multiple risk factors for stroke (e.g., high blood pressure, atrial fibrillation, smoking), compared to that of a young healthy person. Strokes involving the brain stem or cerebellum often cause severe vertigo and imbalance, but nearly always there are other neurological symptoms, such as loss of vision or double vision, numbness or weakness of the face, slurring of speech, and incoordination of one or more limbs. The only stroke that can truly mimic vestibular neuritis is an isolated stroke of the cerebellum. In such a case the only symptoms may be vertigo and imbalance. An experienced neurologist should be able to differentiate the two conditions based on the nystagmus features and the result of the head impulse test (see above), however. As noted above, a CT scan of the brain is of little use in ruling out a stroke in a patient with typical symptoms of vestibular neuritis. Often a brain MRI is considered to be the test that most confidently confirms or refutes the diagnosis of stroke. In our experience, though, it is rare among people with classic signs and symptoms of vestibular neuritis for a brain MRI to change the diagnosis. How to most safely evaluate vertigo in the emergency department remains a major area of research investigation.

A vestibular neuritis–like syndrome could mimic a first attack of **Ménière's disease**. With Ménière's disease, however, the symptoms and signs resolve much faster, typically within hours to a day. In contrast, recovery from vestibular neuritis is measured in weeks to months. Also, a diagnosis of Ménière's disease will become clear over time, with repeated attacks. Vestibular neuritis seldom recurs once you recover.

Red Flags

- Prior history of stroke.*
- Associated neurological symptoms including visual loss, double vision, slurring of speech, incoordination, numbness, or weakness.*
- Symptoms don't improve over a few days.*
- Nystagmus and severe imbalance persist for more than a few days.*

*Could be a stroke or **transient ischemic attack (TIA)**. For more information about stroke and TIAs, see chapter 6.

Stroke and Transient Ischemic Attacks

Over the past few days you have had three brief spells of vertigo and double vision, each lasting about five minutes. You now experience persistent vertigo and severe imbalance. You cannot stand up even with support. You can speak, but your speech is slurred and your right hand is clumsy so that you have difficulty dialing the phone for help.

People often ask us whether their dizziness might be due to a stroke or might be a warning of a stroke to come. Anyone at any age can have a stroke, but some groups have a higher risk of stroke than others. So our answer is yes, especially if you are in the age range for stroke (usually over 60) and/or if you have other risk factors for stroke such as high blood pressure and diabetes. But even then stroke is a relatively rare cause for dizziness compared to other, more benign causes. Most strokes result from blockage of an artery depriving part of the brain of its blood supply. This causes infarction, an area of necrosis (cell death) in the brain, which can be extensive, especially if the blood vessel involved is a large one. If the interruption of blood flow is milder, there may be minimal or no damage. These milder events are called **transient ischemic attacks** (TIAs). Sometimes a TIA can be a warning of an impending stroke. Bleeding into the brain can also cause stroke, but the person having this kind of stroke usually has rapidly progressive and multiple neurological symptoms, including impaired consciousness or loss of consciousness. The symptoms of such a stroke would rarely be confused with the symptoms of other benign causes of dizziness.

Vertigo typically results from interruption of normal blood flow to the brain stem and cerebellum, supplied by the vertebral and basilar arteries. The two vertebral arteries run up the back of the neck and join together at the base of the brain to form the basilar artery, which runs along the brain stem to supply the brain stem and cerebellum (figure 4). Low blood flow in this **vertebrobasilar** artery system commonly causes vertigo and imbalance. This is because the vertebrobasilar artery system supplies brain stem and cerebellar areas that are critical for normal balance. It also supplies blood to both inner ears. By contrast, vertigo does not result from blockage of the carotid arteries, the arteries that run up the front of the neck and supply most of the cerebral cortex and the retina of both eyes. Typical symptoms of carotid artery disease include one-sided visual loss, impaired speech and language, and weakness and numbness on one side of the face and body.

A question that has plagued neurologists for more than a century is whether vertigo and imbalance can be the only symptoms of a vertebrobasilar stroke and TIA or whether there should always be other associated neurological symptoms. After all, the brain stem is packed with critical centers for controlling eye movements, balance, face and body sensation, and coordinated hand and leg movements. Insufficient blood flow to the brain stem should result in a list of neurological symptoms, not just dizziness. It nearly always does. In fact there is a general dictum in neurology that isolated vertigo without other associated neurological symptoms indicates a peripheral vestibular cause—in other words, isolated vertigo

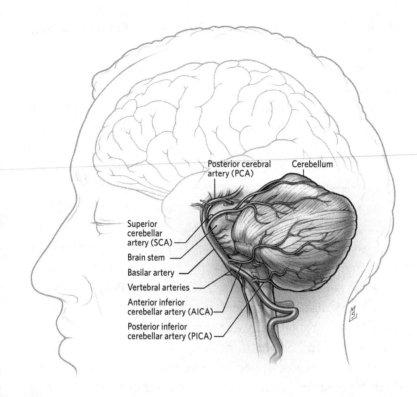

Figure 4 The arterial circulation to the brain stem and cerebellum. The two vertebral arteries join together to form the basilar artery. The main branches are the posterior inferior cerebellar artery (PICA), the anterior inferior cerebellar artery (AICA), the superior cerebellar artery (SCA), and the posterior cerebral artery (PCA). See text for details.

must originate from damage to the inner ear or vestibular nerve. There are exceptions to the rule, however, and in recent years it has become clear that vertigo and imbalance are sometimes the only symptoms of TIA or stroke associated with decreased blood flow within the vertebrobasilar system, particularly when the decreased blood flow selectively involves the cerebellum. But the rare exceptions to the dictum do not negate the concept behind it. Vertigo originating from damage to the brain is nearly always part of a package of other neurological symptoms.

Two major categories of arterial blockage cause stroke: **thrombotic** and **embolic**. With thrombotic stroke, a clot (thrombus) develops in an area of narrowing in the artery; the artery is narrowed because there has been a slow buildup of a cholesterol-laden atherosclerotic plaque in the wall of the artery. A thrombus can occur when the plaque ruptures, exposing deeper layers of the plaque-containing molecules that encourage clotting. This ultimately blocks the artery so blood can no longer flow in it. With embolic stroke, by contrast, debris from a clot breaks loose from the heart or large arteries. It then makes its way to a location downstream in the brain where it becomes lodged in a smaller artery. People with certain heart diseases, particularly an irregular heart rhythm called atrial fibrillation, are at high risk for developing embolic stroke. It is important to distinguish between thrombotic stroke and embolic stroke because treatment is different for each type. Atrial fibrillation is sometimes overlooked until a prolonged EKG monitoring study (of which there are now several types) is performed.

TIAs can occur with all stroke mechanisms but are most common with thrombotic arterial occlusion. TIAs can be a warning of an impending stroke as the thrombus progressively occludes the artery, or sometimes there is a spontaneous remission as blood flow in other nearby arteries takes over for the blocked artery (this is called collateral flow). Embolic blood vessel occlusion can cause TIAs if the clots originating in the heart or large arteries are tiny or if a large clot breaks up into multiple tiny clots when it enters the brain. Each recurrent embolic TIA will have different symptoms depending on which artery or arteries the clots randomly enter and block. By contrast, each TIA resulting from thrombotic vascular occlusion tends to have similar symptoms because the decreased blood flow is always in the same artery.

Typical Symptoms of TIA and Stroke in the Vertebrobasilar System

The best doctors are experts in pattern recognition. They can rapidly make a diagnosis based on the characteristic pattern of symptoms and signs associated with a specific disorder. Nowhere in medicine is this skill more valuable than in diagnosing the different stroke and TIA patterns associated with disease of the vertebrobasilar arteries. Each branch artery supplies a distinct portion of the brain stem and cerebellum, so decreased blood flow in that branch causes a unique combination of symptoms and signs. Vertigo, nystagmus, and imbalance are common with nearly all of the branch artery syndromes, since vestibular pathways run throughout the brain stem and cerebellum. Other more specific associated symptoms and signs define each branch artery syndrome.

A common stroke syndrome associated with vertigo is the Wallenberg syndrome (also called PICA syndrome) resulting from decreased blood flow either in the vertebral artery or in the **posterior inferior cerebellar artery (PICA)** branch, which leaves the vertebral arteries just before they join together to form the basilar artery (see figure 4). Adolf Wallenberg was a German neurologist who described the characteristic signs and symptoms and confirmed the changes via pathology at the end of the nineteenth century. Wallenberg wasn't the first to describe the syndrome bearing his name. A Swiss doctor, Gaspard Vieusseux, detailed the typical symptom complex in 1808, but he did not have pathological confirmation of the stroke location. In addition to vertigo, nystagmus, and imbalance, people who have Wallenberg syndrome (PICA syndrome) experience slurred speech, double vision, and numbness and weakness of the face and extremities. If you look in a mirror you might notice weakness of one side of the face and a small pupil on the same side as the stroke. Hiccups can be unrelenting and pneumonia may develop because impaired swallowing is allowing ingested material to enter the lungs.

Wallenberg syndrome is atypical among stroke syndromes in that it has a higher incidence of occurring in young people with no obvious vascular risk factors. A sudden violent rotation of the neck that may happen during exercise such as weight lifting or with chiropractic manipulation can cause a tear of the vertebral artery in the neck. This can expose deeper layers of the artery wall and produce a clot that eventually breaks loose and enters the PICA or blocks the vertebral artery just before the PICA branch, causing a stroke. The first symptom is often neck pain on the side of the tear for a day or so before the typical symptoms and signs of Wallenberg syndrome begin. Remarkably, most young people with Wallenberg syndrome show relatively good recovery over time, although they usually have some residual symptoms. Rarely, vertigo and imbalance can be the only symptoms of PICA stroke if a small clot originating upstream at the heart or large arteries enters the PICA and becomes lodged in the terminal arteries supplying the cerebellum (sparing the brain stem).

Another vertebrobasilar branch artery syndrome is the AICA (anterior inferior cerebellar artery) syndrome. One of the AICA branches supplies the inner ear. Strokes and TIAs involving the AICA may have both inner ear and brain symptoms and signs, including hearing loss (which otherwise almost never occurs with stroke). Brain symptoms of AICA stroke overlap those of Wallenberg syndrome, although the most common symptom is severe incoordination of the limbs on the side of the blocked artery. Vertigo and hearing loss can be the only symptoms when only the inner ear is involved. In this case, AICA syndrome might be confused with labyrinthitis.

In addition to the characteristic combination of symptoms, the hallmark of TIA and stroke is the sudden onset. The best doctors have a feel for the tempo of symptoms the way a jazz musician has a feel for rhythm. A weak arm that has been getting weaker for two years is not a stroke. Similarly, recurrent dizziness for months is not a stroke. But the sudden onset of vertigo might be a stroke, particularly if there are other neurological symptoms. Stroke and TIA symptoms come on rapidly over minutes; in the case of TIA they can stop abruptly. Ancient Greek doctors used the term "apoplexia," meaning "to cripple by a stroke"; this term emphasizes the sudden catastrophic nature of the symptoms.

CASE EXAMPLE: It's All about Timing

Bill is a 78-year-old retired construction worker with hypertension and diabetes. He was relaxing watching the Steelers play the Cowboys on *Monday Night Football* when he suddenly noted a loud ringing sound in his right ear and felt like the room was spinning. He tried to get up but could not walk. He had a phone in his pocket, and he called 911, with difficulty because his right hand was uncoordinated. When paramedics arrived at his home, his blood pressure was 190/100, and Bill told them he felt numbness of the right side of his face. He was brought to an emergency room, where his blood pressure had improved to 180/80. By the time he saw a doctor, all of his symptoms had resolved. A neurological examination was completely normal. In addition to medications for high blood pressure and diabetes, Bill had been taking one low-dose aspirin tablet every day as a preventative for heart attack and stroke, but he had stopped the aspirin three days earlier because of a nosebleed. Routine blood tests showed only some mild dehydration. The emergency doctor ordered a CT scan of the brain, which was normal, but he was concerned about Bill's report of incoordination of the right hand and numbness of his face, so he decided to admit him to the hospital for further evaluation by a neurologist and for an MRI of the brain. He started an IV to improve hydration, gave him an extra dose of blood pressure medication, and restarted the low-dose aspirin.

During the night his symptoms recurred, and a neurologist was called in from home. When she examined Bill two hours later, she noted a prominent nystagmus and severe imbalance. He could not stand even with support. He had decreased hearing in the right ear, numbness of the face on the right side, and lack of coordination of the right hand. She suspected a brain stem stroke and ordered an emergency MRI of the brain, which was finally completed three hours later, after the technician was called in from home. The radiologist on call reported a small area of infarction involving the right pons (mid portion of the brain stem) consistent with a stroke in the right AICA vascular territory. MRA, a specialized type of MRI that visualizes the arteries, showed narrowing of both vertebral arteries at the junction with the basilar artery. The AICA on the right was blocked shortly after it branched from the basilar artery. The neurologist concluded that Bill had a completed stroke and that there was little to be done at this point, more than five hours after it occurred.

It is hard to find fault with anyone involved in this case. The ER doctor was appropriately concerned about Bill's symptoms, and he restarted aspirin and made sure Bill was hydrated. The neurologist identified the important findings on examination and suspected a brain stem stroke, and the radiologist identified the brain stem stroke and occlusion of the AICA. But as the saying goes, "It's too late to close the barn door once the horse is gone." It was the system that let Bill down.

This scenario plays out regularly at hospitals and emergency rooms around the country, and in fact around the world. Because of the overall dismal track record for treating acute strokes, most major medical centers in the United States have set up acute stroke teams that work with emergency doctors to diagnose and treat stroke patients. Successful treatment of stroke is all about rapid diagnosis and treatment. Literally every minute counts. Time is brain. The old pattern of admitting the patient to the hospital for a leisurely work-up is no longer acceptable. Patients who come to the ER presenting TIA or early stroke require immediate testing to determine the cause; that way treatment can be tailored to the mechanism to prevent a completed stroke. The highest risk of stroke is within 24 hours after a first TIA. A patient who has had several TIAs over several weeks actually has a much lower risk of a stroke. As noted in chapter 5, some major medical centers have set up telestroke programs, using cameras to communicate with rural hospitals and improving the level of care for stroke patients. At UCLA there have been efforts recently to train paramedics to begin stroke treatment on the way to the hospital. Although treatment in the field by paramedics has not yet resulted in improved stroke outcomes, it remains a promising approach.

What Can I Do to Help My Doctor Make the Diagnosis of TIA and Stroke?

The simple answer is to get to a major medical center as fast as possible if you experience symptoms that might be due to a TIA or stroke. It is critical to identify all of the little seemingly unimportant neurological symptoms that occur within the attack. If you experience the sudden onset of dizziness, pay close attention to whether you have other symptoms. In particular, be alert for changes in your vision; facial numbness or tingling; weakness of your face, arm, or leg; trouble speaking or swallowing; and inability to walk. Write down instances in which you have had any of these symptoms during the past several months. If you have a recurring pattern of multiple neurological symptoms in addition to dizziness, this pattern will mean something very different to your doctor than episodes of dizziness alone.

Stopping an antiplatelet or blood-thinning drug such as aspirin can precipitate a TIA or stroke, so it is important to give your doctor details about medications that you have recently stopped. The duration and onset of symptoms is critical for making a correct diagnosis. TIAs start abruptly and typically last minutes. Try to get a clear idea of how often your attacks occur and how long each attack lasts.

What Laboratory Tests Should My Doctor Order and Why?

MRI (magnetic resonance image) and MRA (magnetic resonance angiogram) are the gold standards for diagnosing TIA and stroke. As noted above, routine CT scans of the brain are of little use for identifying small strokes involving the brain stem but can be helpful for ruling out bleeding into the brain, particularly if the doctor is considering treatment to dissolve or retrieve the clot (see below). MRI can identify small strokes in the brain stem and indicate whether the stroke is new or old. MRA can identify the blocked artery and often suggest the likely mechanism for the blockage. The quality of MRA images has improved as MRI technology has improved, but the resolution of MRA is still limited to imaging larger arteries.

CT angiography (CTA) is another rapidly improving non-invasive technique for visualizing brain arteries, and it often has better resolution than MRA. CTA uses x-rays, so it isn't done on everyone, but in an emergency it can provide high-quality information. Sometimes, conventional catheter angiography is required, particularly if more aggressive intervention such as clot retrieval is being considered. With this procedure a catheter is inserted in an artery, typically in the thigh, and guided to the brain arteries of interest where a small amount of contrast dye is released. This technique allows excellent visualization of the artery and its branches. Once the area of blockage is clearly identified, a clot-retrieval device in the catheter can grab the clot and vacuum or mechanically drag it out of the blocked artery.

If there is no obvious explanation for the stroke on MRA or CT angiography, then your doctor will focus on the heart as a source of emboli (clots). A routine EKG and blood tests to rule out a heart attack should be performed, since embolic strokes are common after heart attacks. Ultrasound studies of the heart (echocardiograms) can often identify the source of emboli in the heart or large vessels leaving the heart. A more prolonged EKG monitoring for days with a so-called Holter monitor—basically an EKG with a computer that you wear around for a period of days to record your heart rhythm—may be necessary to identify intermittent heart arrhythmias such as atrial fibrillation, which is strongly associated with intermittent emboli to the brain. Holter monitor studies usually last 24 to 48 hours, and cardiologists use various devices to make longer recordings, sometimes lasting months.

What Is the Best Treatment for TIA and Stroke?

The best treatment of TIA and stroke depends on what's causing the arterial blockage. To some extent, as with everything else, it depends what works in the individual. Most TIAs result from sudden blockage of an artery by a clot. Antiplatelet drugs such as aspirin or clopidogrel (Plavix) are commonly the first line of treatment. These drugs prevent platelets from aggregating (sticking together) and contributing to blood clots in arteries damaged by cholesterol plaques. These medications decrease the risk that a TIA will evolve into a stroke. If your blood tests have shown an elevated blood level of cholesterol, or LDL, lipid-lowering medications (statins) will also decrease the risk of TIA and stroke. Sometimes TIAs recur or strokes develop even though a patient is taking antiplatelet drugs and statins, particularly when the patient has a high-grade blockage, such as in Bill's case described above. In this case anticoagulants should be considered. These drugs interfere with clot formation and can even partially dissolve fresh clots. There is general agreement that most patients with known atrial fibrillation should be treated with a daily anticoagulant medication because of the high risk for developing brain emboli and stroke.

One of the major recent advancements in stroke treatment is the use of intravenous (IV) tissue plasminogen activator (tPA) to dissolve the clot causing the stroke. It has been estimated that in at least one-third of cases, IV tPA will dissolve the clot and reverse symptoms and signs. The sooner the drug is given after stroke onset, the higher the likelihood for success. Current guidelines recommend giving IV tPA only during the first three hours after stroke onset (sometimes a little more, depending on individual characteristics), and the earlier the better. This explains the need for rapid diagnosis. IV tPA should in most cases be used according to nationally accepted guidelines intended to balance the benefit of reversing a stroke with the risk of brain hemorrhage. These guidelines are in constant flux, as technology improves and new technologies are invented. You should find out which hospital near you is best equipped to treat stroke, as many communities have one or more designated stroke centers with extra expertise in management of complex stroke scenarios; if you have a stroke, you and your family will then know which hospital you should ideally be rushed to.

Clot retrieval with a catheter device, as described above, is another dramatic new treatment technique for treating acute stroke. Again, this technique only works with fresh clots, so timing is critical. One of the most devastating stroke syndromes involving the vertebrobasilar system is occlusion of the basilar artery with a clot. With "locked in syndrome" the patient is fully alert but cannot make any movement and cannot speak. Although risky, clot retrieval can lead to a dramatic cure.

What Can I Do on My Own to Treat TIA and Stroke?

The short answer is to call 911. The faster you can get to an emergency room, preferably one at a stroke center with an acute stroke team, the greater the chances are that your symptoms will be successfully treated. What can you do while waiting for the ambulance? Two simple things may help: lie flat with your legs elevated to improve circulation to the brain and drink fluids to improve hydration. Should you take an aspirin tablet? Usually yes, although this is not without some risk. The potential benefits usually exceed the risks, as 80 to 90 percent of strokes are caused by arterial blockage and only 10 to 20 percent by bleeding in the brain. If the symptoms include worst headache ever or altered consciousness, then you should *not* take an aspirin, since the chance that the stroke is due to bleeding into the brain is greater.

TIA and Stroke Mimics

Most **epileptic seizures** include sudden loss of consciousness or profoundly altered consciousness. These types of symptoms tend to be easily recognized by a neurologist, and they are less common with TIA. Some types of seizures, such as focal motor seizures that involve shaking of a limb followed by paralysis, can be confused with TIA because they may cause weakness of one part of the body and do not include loss of consciousness, but these seizures tend to be much shorter than TIA—lasting only a minute or so. **Migraine with aura**—previously called complicated migraine—can cause episodes of dizziness along with many other neurological symptoms, including numbness or weakness on one side of the face or body. Usually these episodes are associated with other migraine symptoms such as headache and light and sound sensitivity, but occasionally they occur without other migraine symptoms. Most people with this pattern will have had typical migraine headaches or visual aura in the past and have a family history of migraine. One should think of migraine when a person with TIA-like episodes has normal MRI and MRA and normal heart studies. (See chapter 4 for more information about migraine syndromes.)

When a person goes to the emergency room because of prolonged severe vertigo and imbalance and does not have any other symptoms, the main concern is whether or not it could be a stroke. Statistically, this presentation is much more likely to be **vestibular neuritis**. To a trained neurologist the only stroke syndrome that can truly mimic vestibular neuritis is an isolated stroke of the cerebellum. As mentioned in chapter 5, doctors can reliably distinguish between these two possibilities during a neurological examination. The gold standard for diagnosing stroke is usually MRI of the brain, though it must be said that no one test is infallible. Several autoimmune and genetic disorders can cause multiple arterial blockages producing TIAs and strokes. These conditions tend to occur in younger people and to be rapidly progressive, with multiple strokes occurring over a short period of time.

Red Flags

- Dizziness with severe weakness and numbness below the neck. Could be warning of impending occlusion of the basilar artery.
- Dizziness with worst ever headache. Could be hemorrhage into brain stem or cerebellum.
- Dizziness with severe imbalance so that you cannot stand even with support. Could be cerebellar infarct.
- Loss of consciousness after stroke-like episode. Could reflect potentially fatal brain swelling caused by infarction.

**PART IV   CONSTANT DIZZINESS THAT LASTS
24 HOURS A DAY FOR MONTHS AND
EVEN YEARS**

CHAPTER 7

Dizziness and Anxiety

You have been constantly dizzy for eight months. The dizziness takes several forms, from a lightheaded, swimming sensation to a sense of spinning inside the head even as your surroundings remain still. At times you have the bizarre sensation that the floor is moving up toward you or that you may fall even when you are sitting still in a chair. You have had occasional dizziness in the past—lasting a month or two—but never this severe for this long. You have always been an anxious person, and you had a few panic attacks when you were younger, but the anxiety seems to have gotten much worse since this constant dizziness started.

People with an anxiety disorder typically do not go to doctors complaining of **anxiety**. Instead, they complain of other symptoms, including dizziness, palpitations, headache, gastrointestinal symptoms, and cognitive impairment. In studies of anxiety-related symptoms, dizziness is by far the most common, occurring in about two-thirds of those who have anxiety. Anxiety-related dizziness has been given many names, including chronic subjective dizziness, psychophysiological dizziness, and phobic dizziness. These are vague terms that are not very satisfying to patients or doctors.

Anxiety is a negative emotion experienced in anticipation of a real or imagined threat or dangerous circumstances.

Nearly everyone experiences mild anxiety from time to time, but some people have an anxiety diathesis, meaning that they have an above-average emotional and physical response to threats. When an anxiety diathesis becomes severe enough to interfere with how someone functions in the world, the person is said to have an anxiety disorder. Most people with anxiety disorder have a family member with anxiety. Recent genetic studies have identified specific genetic variations that make it more likely that a person will develop anxiety disorder. But how these genetic variations lead to dizziness and other symptoms is largely unknown.

Looking at the matter from another point of view, many people with dizziness also have an anxiety diathesis. A considerable proportion of these people could be diagnosed with anxiety disorder. Many patients in our clinics do not have a past history of an anxiety disorder that preceded the onset of dizziness, however. It can therefore be difficult or impossible to know whether an anxiety disorder is causing dizziness or some other disorder that causes dizziness, such as an inner ear disorder, is also causing anxiety. As some people with dizziness say, "I was never anxious, until I started feeling dizzy."

Indeed, based on data from the US Census Bureau's 2008 National Health Interview Survey, one study found that people with "vestibular vertigo" were three times more likely to have depression, anxiety, and/or panic disorder. Vestibular vertigo was defined as spinning vertigo, positional vertigo, or recurrent dizziness and nausea with either movement of the visual scene or with head movement or imbalance. Although such an association study does not establish a cause-and-effect relationship between dizziness and anxiety and depression, it does indicate that if you are dizzy, you are more likely to have anxiety and depression than the general population. Can we say whether the psychiatric symptoms or the vestibular vertigo came first in an individual patient? Often we cannot. A practical approach is to take the view that anxiety and dizziness often co-occur, and both need to be addressed, either with the same intervention or with separate interventions.

Discussing which genes are involved in the risk for anxiety disorder is beyond the scope of this book, but there is scientific agreement that multiple genes are involved. Some genes increase the risk of developing anxiety disorder while others decrease it. Variations in genes associated with the production and breakdown of the neurotransmitter serotonin have received great attention because medications that raise the serotonin level in the brain have proven effective in treating anxiety. However, there is little doubt that variations in many other genes eventually will be identified as contributing to the production of anxiety disorder. The availability of the human genome and rapid, cost-efficient gene sequencing have accelerated the pace of genetic research. Unexpected links are being found between psychiatric disorders previously thought to be distinct and unrelated. Such disorders are likely to be substantially reclassified in the near future using genetic criteria.

What happens when a person who is already predisposed to anxiety disorder develops BPPV? The person may avoid seeking medical help because of fear of experiencing vertigo in the course of diagnosis and treatment. After all, the only way to diagnose and treat BPPV is to go through position changes, lying down and sitting up, which will inevitably cause a recurrence of vertigo. The person with BPPV may therefore avoid seeing a doctor or physical therapist, despite knowing full well that getting medical help is the only route to a cure.

When people with anxiety disorder develop inner ear damage, such as with vestibular neuritis, it may take longer than expected for them to recover. With respect to such recovery, it should be noted that no one really knows in detail what factors influence recovery from vestibular neuritis, although vestibular suppressant medications such as meclizine slow down recovery and vestibular physical therapy helps recovery. Nevertheless, the concept that genetically determined anxiety traits adversely affect recovery from vestibular disorders is consistent with both the medical literature and our clinical experience. In the future, it may become routine to treat brain chemical disorders such as anxiety disorders as part of a comprehensive approach to rehabilitation after vestibular damage, such as occurs with vestibular neuritis. This is somewhat analogous to treating post-stroke depression as part of a comprehensive approach to rehabilitation after stroke—a principle on which there is some consensus among neurologists.

But why might a person with anxiety have more difficulty recovering from a vestibular disorder? Could the person who is anxious be unable to concentrate on or fully participate in rehabilitation exercises, resulting in less than optimal completion of such exercises? Or could the problem in compensation be some deeper physiological connection between anxiety, dizziness, and spatial orientation? One fascinating aspect of this question is the concept of excessive visual dependence. The brain relies on the different senses to varying degrees. If the brain perceives that one sense is more reliable than another, the less reliable sense will be ignored, and the brain will rely to a greater extent on information from the "good" (i.e., more reliable) senses. When a person is in the early stages of vestibular neuritis, the information the brain receives from the inner ears is faulty and unreliable. The brain knows it can't depend on the inner ears for accurate guidance on position and motion, at least until it figures out what to do with the confusing asymmetric signals it is receiving. Eventually, the brain will compensate and learn how to balance the signals from the two ears. So what does it do in the meantime? It relies on vision and other senses to a greater than normal degree. This strategy, while highly useful, may also have dysfunctional consequences. Complex visual environments like a grocery store become overwhelming. Walking down the aisle of a store may be akin to an amusement park ride.

It has been hypothesized that the problem of maladaptive or excessive visual dependence is more common in people who, at baseline, rely greatly on vision for balance. Do such people exist? In fact, there is a range of normal extent of visual dependence. However, it has been found that people with anxiety disorder rely more than other people on vision. In one study, people with an anxiety disorder who viewed large projections of moving video patterns exhibited greater body sway than average. They appeared to interpret the movement of the projection as real movement of the Earth. Once we have a better understanding of how to manipulate visual dependence, we may be able to help people with dizziness to return to visually complex environments such as that bright, crowded grocery store. Furthermore, it is likely that such vision-based interventions will be particularly helpful for the subset of people who have both a vestibular disorder and anxiety.

Is there a relationship between anxiety disorder and migraine? Yes, about 50 percent of families with migraine have anxiety disorder coexisting in affected family members. There are clearly overlapping genetic susceptibility factors for anxiety disorder and migraine. Because dizziness is common with both disorders, being aware of their coexistence can be important for developing treatment strategies (see below).

Typical Symptoms of Anxiety Disorders?

The *Diagnostic and Statistical Manual of Mental Disorders* (DSM), published by the American Psychiatric Association, for many years has provided consensus criteria for the diagnosis of psychiatric disorders. This is a diagnostic handbook that allows one to make a confident diagnosis of a broad range of conditions, including major depressive disorder, generalized anxiety disorder, and many other common and uncommon psychological problems. There are several common anxiety disorders, including generalized anxiety disorder (anxiety most of the time), obsessive-compulsive disorder (associated with frequent intrusive thoughts and the need to perform certain behaviors that make no sense but temporarily alleviate discomfort), post-traumatic stress disorder (anxiety related to a particular set of traumatic events), social phobia (prominent avoidance of interaction with people), and panic disorder (recurrent attacks of anxiety). The DSM provides a framework within which doctors can agree on a working diagnosis and a best approach to treatment. However, there are limitations on how much the DSM can tell us.

We are in desperate need of biomarkers for anxiety disorder. A biomarker may be defined as any objective and reproducible measurement that serves as an indicator of normal physiology or disease activity. In other words, we need something to measure that is more objective and reliable than simply asking people, "Are you anxious?" or "How anxious are you?" A genetic test would be ideal. Or a brain scan. Or possibly a physiological measurement of vision or balance that includes motion of the visual scene. In the practice of medicine, biomarkers allow reliable observations that contribute to an intelligent diagnosis. For example, if you have diabetes, your doctor will order a blood test called the hemoglobin A1C test to track your sugar control. If you have hypertension, your doctor will track your blood pressure. And if you have heart disease, your doctor may monitor a heart ultrasound number called the ejection fraction, which quantifies the amount of blood your heart can pump.

We foresee that in the future, rather than using diagnoses based on the DSM, doctors will instead say something like, "You have a gene that affects how much calcium flows into brain cells"—or "You have a neurotransmitter receptor that is slightly less responsive than average"—"and as a result, you have symptoms, including persistent dizziness, depressed mood, panic attacks, chronic low-level anxiety, and some tendency toward having obsessions and compulsions." In other words, we expect that genetic research will help clarify the molecular basis of psychiatric disorders, including those that cause dizziness. We look forward to a day when a person with dizziness might take a simple blood test and the doctor will be able to identify at least some biological markers as contributors to dizziness. This will assist doctors in selecting the best therapies, much as oncologists can now do selection of chemotherapy medications based on the genetic characteristics of particular cancers.

CASE EXAMPLE: I've Had a Lot of Tests, but the Doctors Don't Know What's Wrong

John is a 45-year-old editor who has been experiencing dizziness constantly for the past two years. The dizziness is difficult to describe. It's a sensation inside his head that is somewhere between swimming and spinning. He has sudden "earthquake"-like sensations where he will grab onto nearby objects—though he has never fallen. He feels unsteady on his feet even though he still plays golf the same as always and is one of the better bowlers on the company team. He has had a head CT, a brain MRI, an EEG, a VNG with caloric tests, a hearing test, an EKG and an exercise treadmill test, a panel of blood work, and a nerve-conduction study, all of which have been normal. He almost wishes someone would find something serious so at least they could put a label on his disease. Each new doctor brings up a list of suggestions of possible serious illnesses, suggestions that make him feel even worse. He is also under a lot of stress at work and at home. He works long hours, and his boss is very demanding. He has three teenage daughters. His mother lives in a nursing home, and he is her only child.

John's dizziness is present when he wakes up in the morning, and it's still there when he goes to bed at night. Recently he had not been sleeping well, and his doctor gave him a prescription for alprazolam (Xanax) that helped some. Last year, after a busy period at work, his family took a vacation, and he was surprised to find that his dizziness improved after daily walks on the beach. Many years ago he had a handful of panic attacks, but none recently. He has always been an anxious person, but he feels that his anxiety has markedly increased since the dizziness started two years ago. His mother has also had panic attacks and is currently receiving medications for anxiety disorder.

We see several patients like John in our clinics on a weekly basis. One feature they all tend to have in common is their frustration with doctors and the medical system overall. They invariably have been referred to different specialists who have ordered multiple tests within their specialty. Each subspecialist "feels the elephant" from her particular perspective and usually decides the problem does not reside in the area of her subspecialty. Although the tests usually come back normal, an occasional borderline abnormality or an unrelated incidental finding leads to a spurt of new anxiety and a transient worsening of symptoms.

What John needs is reassurance, one of the most ancient of doctors' healing powers. The "vicious cycle" nature of anxiety disorder cannot be overemphasized. The symptoms are real and not imagined, and there is an interrelationship between the dizziness and anxiety. Both result from an underlying neurochemical disorder. Concerns that the dizziness may be a symptom of a more ominous disorder such as brain tumor or multiple sclerosis markedly increase anxiety and dizziness.

What Can I Do to Help My Doctor Make the Diagnosis of Anxiety-related Dizziness?

Many people with this problem will have had anxiety in the past. It is important to let your doctor know if you have previously noted anxiety symptoms, even if they occurred many years ago. Did you have a series of panic attacks as a teenager? Have you always had a difficult time relaxing? Have you been treated for anxiety or depression in the past?

Try to identify situations that increase or decrease your symptoms. For some medical problems, exercise can aggravate symptoms, but for people with anxiety, it often does just the opposite. Exercise helps, and avoiding exercise leads to an increase in anxiety. If it's been a long time since you exercised, the dizziness may initially be worse, so you will need to gradually increase your exercise level. Conversely, the new emergence of anxiety may be linked to a decrease in exercise related to an illness, new job, or other life events. For many people with anxiety-related dizziness, the symptoms just occur under certain conditions. Situations that might induce anxiety-related dizziness include thinking about one's illness or that of family members, a new job with increased responsibilities, and driving on the freeway.

The diagnosis of an illness can sometimes be aided by the response to medications. This strategy is called pharmacologic dissection. For example, if someone responds to a class of headache medication called triptans, such as sumatriptan (Imitrex) or rizatriptan (Maxalt), then that person is considered to likely have migraine. This approach is attractive because it probes biology in specific ways and at the same time gives information about which interventions work to help people. It can be helpful for your doctor to know whether your dizziness improved during a trial of any of the medications that help anxiety, particularly a selective serotonin reuptake inhibitor such as fluoxetine (Prozac) or citalopram (Celexa) or a tricyclic amine such as amitriptyline (Elavil) or nortriptyline (Pamelor). Because of the genetic nature of anxiety disorders, it is helpful to know if a family member has anxiety disorder and has responded well to a particular medication.

What Laboratory Tests Should My Doctor Order and Why?

Because there are no biomarkers for disorders involving anxiety, there is no laboratory test that is specific for anxiety disorder. A detailed medical history and examination are the only things required to make the diagnosis. Although laboratory tests may be useful to rule out other causes of dizziness, there is a risk that the tests and the results might be triggers for worsening anxiety and dizziness.

What Is the Best Treatment for Anxiety-related Dizziness?

A discussion of the best treatment for anxiety-related dizziness must address two groups of people. Those in the first group have no significant contributor to dizziness other than the anxiety disorder. Those in the second may or may not have a preexisting anxiety disorder but have developed severe anxiety in the setting of another cause of dizziness, such as vestibular neuritis, Ménière's disease, or BPPV.

Treatment of those for whom an anxiety disorder appears to be the primary cause of dizziness most often consists of a combination of nonpharmacological and pharmacological interventions. Nonpharmacological interventions include exercise, meditation, yoga, counseling, and psychotherapy. Pharmacological interventions may include selective serotonin reuptake inhibitors (such as sertraline, citalopram, escitalopram), tricyclic amines (nortriptyline, amitriptyline), and/or benzodiazepines (clonazepam, alprazolam, lorazepam). Benzodiazepines should not be used on a daily basis for long periods of time because people taking these drugs develop a tolerance for them and dependence on them.

The treatment of those for whom a vestibular disorder has triggered or greatly exacerbated anxiety should combine the approaches used for treatment of anxiety in general with therapies for the underlying vestibular disorder. In addition, some attention should be given to whether a person has developed excessive visual dependence. If so, it may be possible to address his visual dependence with vestibular physical therapy. Some physical therapists think that excessive visual dependence can be helped by exercises that train people to use their other senses, particularly the sensations from the limbs and body, called somatosensory input. Unfortunately there have been no controlled treatment trials for this type of therapy, so it is unclear whether it is superior to other exercise routines such as yoga.

What Can I Do to Treat Anxiety-related Dizziness?

Three major triggers for anxiety-related symptoms are stress, lack of sleep, and irregular eating patterns with bingeing. Regular exercise is probably the best overall stress management technique. It is good for overall health and also helps with sleep. As a rule, regular use of sleeping pills should be avoided since all are associated with development of tolerance and dependence. Some people benefit from melatonin taken on a regular basis to induce natural sleep. Food should be spaced throughout the day with something for breakfast, lunch, and dinner. Moderate use of caffeine, such as in coffee and soft drinks, is usually tolerated, but bingeing one day and withdrawing the next can be a problem. Stimulants such as cocaine can be catastrophic in people with anxiety disorder.

Mindfulness meditation is an increasingly popular approach to addressing anxiety. One simple way to learn about the concepts of mindfulness meditation is to read Herbert Benson's classic, *The Relaxation Response*. You can also ask your doctor about resources for learning about meditation. More and more doctors are incorporating mindfulness meditation into their practices, at least at the level of providing a brief handout. In some geographic areas, doctors are able to refer to resources such as the Benson-Henry Institute for Mind Body Medicine at Massachusetts General Hospital. There are many guided meditation recordings on the Internet. One example is the collection of free guided meditation audio recordings available through the UCLA Mindful Awareness Research Center (http://marc.ucla.edu/body.cfm?id=22).

Mimics of Anxiety-related Dizziness

Anxiety can result from excessive release of endogenous hormones called catecholamines (such as epinephrine, norepinephrine). A rare but serious cause of excessive release of these chemicals is a tumor of the adrenal gland called a **pheochromocytoma**. One clue to diagnosis of a pheochromocytoma is high blood pressure, especially when the high blood pressure comes in waves along with feelings of panic (this occurs when the tumor releases catecholamines). People may have waves of low blood pressure caused by the decrease in levels of catecholamines after these compounds have been released, peaked in level, and then cleared. A common mimic of primary anxiety disorders is dysfunction of the autonomic nervous system, often manifested as the **postural orthostatic tachycardia syndrome (POTS)** (see chapter 2). Many people who have been diagnosed with POTS in their twenties were previously diagnosed with anxiety disorder beginning in their early teenage years or even earlier, suggesting that POTS may be part of a complex anxiety disorder that begins in childhood. Many people with POTS who had childhood anxiety also have a history of repeated fainting during childhood.

The distinction between POTS and an anxiety disorder may be somewhat artificial, but an anxiety disorder is more likely if the person develops autonomic symptoms and signs only once in a while, and POTS is more likely if the autonomic symptoms are present most of the time.

Red Flags

- Chest pain, heart palpitations, and shortness of breath on exertion. Although all of these symptoms could be associated with panic disorder, they could also indicate a heart attack or other cardiovascular or lung issues, particularly in an older person with vascular risk factors.
- Waves of very high blood pressure (>200 systolic). Could indicate the presence of a tumor of the adrenal gland called a pheochromocytoma.
- Episodes of very rapid heart rate (>140 beats per minute). Could be POTS or cardiac arrhythmia.

CHAPTER 8

Mal de Debarquement Syndrome

You return from a cruise ship vacation and find that when you step onto dry land, you feel as if you are still on a rocking ship. You have had this sensation briefly before, so you expect that it will resolve, but it doesn't. You feel unsteady on your feet, but you are able to go on with routine activities. Curiously, you feel best when you are in motion, such as riding in an automobile. Although the symptoms temporarily remit while in motion, they are worse when you stop moving.

Mal de debarquement syndrome (MdDS) is defined by a persistent feeling of motion—usually with an element of slowly rocking from side to side—and a sense of imbalance while walking. MdDS usually occurs after exposure to motion, most commonly on a ship, airplane, or long ride in an automobile. Many people who have sailed on a ship have noted the persistence of a sensation of rocking after disembarking that lasts for minutes to hours. This is usually considered to be a normal phenomenon. For the person with MdDS, though, the rocking sensation may continue for months or even years.

When a person with MdDS is in motion, riding in an automobile, for instance, the rocking sensation temporarily stops. However, once the person leaves the vehicle and is again sitting or standing still, the feeling of rocking returns and is often temporarily worse. For unknown reasons, this disorder is more common in women than in men and is associated with anxiety disorders and migraine. Genetic susceptibility may be an important factor for developing the syndrome. While the exact mechanism of MdDS is unknown, most experts believe this syndrome has something to do with how the brain adapts to motion.

The types of motion one feels on a ship are complex. It is common, for example, for a person standing on the deck of the ship to experience roll to the right and the left combined with heaving up and down. One theory suggests that while on a ship, in a vehicle, or in any situation in which the person is constantly in motion, the brain in some fashion learns to associate feelings of continuous motion with turning of the head from side to side, as when looking off the deck of a ship to search the water for dolphins or turning the head to look around the pool for the snack bar. When a ship passenger returns to land, the brain recalls the previously learned association and produces a feeling of rocking that mimics what was present on the ship. In our modern world the brain is constantly adapting to different motion experiences, and usually it does so with little difficulty. Sometimes it can take a while for the brain to make the adjustment, but eventually it does. However, with MdDS for some reason the brain becomes "stuck" in a constant motion mode.

If a normal person is spun around multiple times on a rotating chair and then suddenly stopped, she will have a persistent after-sensation of rotation that will gradually dwindle. The rate of the decay is defined by a vestibulo-ocular reflex (VOR) time constant, the time it takes for the sensation to decay to 63 percent of the initial magnitude. The signal of rotation is picked up by the semicircular canals in the inner ear and passed on the nerve cells in the brain where reverberating circuits prolong the sensation well beyond the duration of the signal generated in the inner ear (often called velocity storage). The normal VOR time constant can range from 5 to 40 seconds. VOR time constants can be measured by a test your doctor can order called rotational testing in the dark, also known as rotatory chair testing (see chapter 5). It has been suggested that people with longer time constants are more susceptible to MdDS. In other words, overactivity within these reverberating central vestibular pathways may be a factor in developing MdDS. Prolonged repetitive rotations and certain drugs can shorten the time constant and possibly improve MdDS, but so far there have not been any controlled treatment trials using these techniques.

There is a consensus that tests of inner ear function, both auditory and vestibular, are generally normal in patients with MdDS, and scans of the brain do not reveal any abnormalities. Some recent studies using brain positron emission tomography (PET), which measures glucose uptake, and functional MRI, which typically measures oxygen uptake, have found increased resting state metabolic activity and abnormal functional connectivity between areas of the brain that process visual and vestibular signals in patients with MdDS. These findings will need to be replicated in a larger number of patients, but if true they might provide an objective marker for this poorly understood disorder.

What Are the Typical Symptoms of Mal de Debarquement Syndrome?

After returning from a boat, plane, or automobile voyage, or less commonly after exposure to other types of motion, the affected person develops a continuous sense of rocking. The feelings of rocking are combined with a feeling of imbalance that is particularly notable when the person tries to walk. Some have described this as comparable to walking on a trampoline. Sometimes there is mild associated nausea, but it is rarely severe. A key feature of the syndrome is that those suffering it feel much better when back in motion, only to have the symptoms recur when they are again still. Symptoms similar to those of MdDS can sometimes be triggered by visual motion, such as standing on a pier and watching a rough sea. Sometimes symptoms develop spontaneously, without any apparent trigger, in which case there is often an associated anxiety disorder and migraine. People with MdDS often report that the sensation of rocking is less intense when they are preoccupied with daily activities and worst when they are sitting quietly and thinking about the symptoms.

CASE EXAMPLE: I Don't Know What This Is, but You're Fine

Jennifer is a 39-year-old mom. After returning from a cruise with her family, she felt the ground was rocking when she got off the ship. She thought this was normal, but the symptom continued without stopping. She feels unsteady on her feet ("like walking on a trampoline") even though she is able to carry on all normal activities. The rocking sensation is present all the time, whenever she is awake. The only time she feels good is when she is riding in an automobile. When the sensation of rocking persisted for several days off the ship, she saw her primary care doctor, who was baffled and sent her to an otolaryngologist.

The otolaryngologist ordered a hearing test and a videonystagmogram (VNG), both of which were normal, and referred her to a neurologist. The neurologist felt that Jennifer may be suffering from anxiety disorder. He ordered a brain MRI, and when this came back normal, he simply said, "You're fine, don't worry about it." After several more months of continuous rocking sensations, she finally found a doctor who had heard of MdDS. He was supportive but told her there was no known treatment and she would have to live with it.

People with MdDS are often frustrated with how the medical system deals with their syndrome. Few doctors have heard of MdDS, and many of those who have are suspicious that it is a psychiatric disorder. Although there may be some susceptibility factors in common with anxiety disorder, MdDS is remarkably stereotyped, and there is convincing evidence for central nervous system dysfunction.

Unfortunately, it is true that there is no well-established treatment for MdDS at this time, but this may be changing. People with the disorder should follow up regularly with their doctors and can obtain support from patient groups such as the MdDS Balance Disorder Foundation. There are several promising research efforts that offer hope for a cure of this disorder, as described below.

What Can I Do to Help My Doctor Make the Diagnosis of Mal de Debarquement Syndrome?

There are two distinct features of MdDS that effectively make the diagnosis: the symptoms begin after the person has been in motion for a prolonged period, and symptoms are relieved when the person is back in motion, such as in a moving car. In contrast, most other types of dizziness, particularly inner ear disorders, are *aggravated*, not relieved, by motion. If the person has experienced dizziness after prolonged motion in the past, that history can also be helpful in making the diagnosis. The next step may be convincing your doctor that there is such a disorder because many doctors are not familiar with it. The number of articles on MdS in the scientific and lay literature has mushroomed recently, however, so more and more doctors are becoming aware of this syndrome.

What Laboratory Tests Should My Doctor Order and Why?

Most often the answer is none. In tests of hundreds of people with mal de debarquement syndrome, no significant abnormality of inner ear or brain function has been found. People with MdDS feel unsteady on their feet, but they are able to carry on many normal activities and generally do not fall. If you have symptoms that indicate inner ear problems or neurological problems—vertigo, hearing loss, or severe imbalance, for example—then laboratory tests are probably in order.

What Is the Best Treatment?

At this time there is no well-established, widely accepted treatment for MdDS. The good news is that there are some leads on possible treatments. Because MdDS is now conceptualized as a disorder of maladaptive brain plasticity, it makes sense that our standard approach to brain adaptation—namely, physical therapy—might have something to offer. However, no clinical trials have demonstrated the effectiveness of even specialized vestibular physical therapy in the treatment of MdDS. Many patients report that controlled motor activity, such as with yoga or tai chi, helps the symptoms, but it is not clear whether it is the physical activity or the relaxation that is beneficial.

One concept for curing MdDS involves using repetitive stimulation of the vestibular and visual systems to train the brain to stop perceiving motion where there is none. In one procedure recently implemented at a single academic center, patients are treated by rolling the head from side to side while watching a rotating full-field visual stimulus. Seventy percent of patients reported prolonged benefit lasting up to a year, but these results need to be confirmed in controlled treatment trials.

Another type of treatment for MdDS that is under investigation is repetitive transcranial magnetic stimulation (rTMS), a technique in which painless magnetic pulses are applied to the outside of the head to induce electrical currents in the brain. Preliminary studies using brain PET and functional brain MRI to evaluate rTMS in patients with MdDS have shown increased metabolic activity in central visual-vestibular pathways. These findings suggest that the stimulation was well tolerated, and most subjects reported improvement in symptoms. One of the main criticisms of rTMS is that it stimulates a large area of the brain, even with careful targeting of the magnetic pulses, raising questions about whether the brain circuits involved can really be selectively stimulated. There is, however, a growing community of researchers studying rTMS and other forms of electrical stimulation of the brain, all of which hold some potential promise for development of future interventions for the treatment of neurological and psychiatric disorders. Much more work needs to be done and controlled treatment trials must be performed before the effectiveness of this approach can be confirmed; if the rTMS technique is shown to be effective in trials, then the trials will also serve to identify the most effective stimulus settings and locations.

What is the role of medications in treating MdDS? No medication has been consistently effective in stopping the symptoms. Some patients report improvement with benzodiazepines such as diazepam or clonazepam, which should ideally be limited to intermittent use for "bad days" because these medications can cause tolerance and dependency. Antidepressant drugs such as the tricyclic amines (amitriptyline, nortriptyline) and selective serotonin reuptake inhibitors (fluoxetine, citalopram) have been helpful in some patients, but it is unclear whether the benefit comes from relief of anxiety and depression or from another effect on the vestibular system. However, it really doesn't matter, as long as the intervention alleviates the symptoms. Controlled clinical trials of medications for MdDS are needed, as for the other proposed physical and device-based methods of MdDS treatment. Another aspect of medication use has to do with whether one can prevent recurrence of MdDS symptoms by taking a benzodiazepine medication such as clonazepam during exposure to provocative motion, such as with prolonged air travel. This seems to be a helpful strategy, though its benefit remains to be tested in controlled trials.

What Can I Do on My Own to Treat Mal de Debarquement?

Many people with MdDS report that controlled exercise routines such as yoga and tai chi can provide some relief of symptoms. Clearly, people with MdDS who are sedentary do worse than those who participate in a regular exercise routine. Ruminating about the symptoms makes them worse. Meditation and other relaxation techniques are helpful for some people. So-called cognitive therapy attempts to distract the person from dwelling on the continuous motion sensation.

Obviously, it is essential to have the correct diagnosis. Many people in our clinics have been told they have MdDS when in fact they have something completely different—and treatable. Lastly, you need to stay informed of new developments in the treatment of this disorder. There is research going on now that may greatly affect how this disorder will be treated in just a few years. Online materials from the MdDS Balance Disorder Foundation and the Vestibular Disorders Association (VEDA) have increased awareness of the disorder through patients' stories and information about ongoing research.

Mal de Debarquement Mimics

Occasionally, doctors will confuse MdDS and **motion sickness**, which is understandable since both are perturbations of brain function induced by exposure to motion. Indeed, motion sickness and MdDS may have some mechanisms in common, and ultimately the treatments for both may prove to be similar. At this time, the main distinction is that the person with motion sickness feels worst during exposure to motion and improves once the exposure to motion ceases. In contrast, the person with MdDS generally feels normal or improves during exposure to motion and notes onset or increase in symptoms when the motion ceases.

By far the dizziness syndrome most commonly confused with MdDS is the dizziness associated with anxiety disorders and migraine. As noted above, sometimes MdDS symptoms spontaneously develop in people who have anxiety disorder and migraine. Whether spontaneous and classic MdDS (developing after a motion experience) are the same or different phenomena is currently unclear. This is an important question to answer, since treatments may be different for spontaneous and post-motion-exposure MdDS. Complicating matters further, patients with anxiety disorders and migraine often describe a rocking sensation but not the other characteristic features of MdDS. The rocking sensations perceived by some people with migraine are usually less persistent than what people with MdDS feel, though of course it is possible to have both disorders. Much more research is needed to address these questions.

Red Flags

- Severe imbalance, with falling. May suggest a neurological disorder such as cerebellar ataxia or other brain or spinal cord disorders.
- Visual surroundings are unstable when the head is in motion (oscillopsia). May indicate loss of vestibular function on both sides (see chapter 9).
- Rocking sensation becomes worse when in motion. May be an inner ear disorder.

Dizziness Due to Loss of Vestibular Function in Both Ears

You have had several spells of vertigo in the past, but now you are constantly dizzy and off balance. When you walk, the area in front of you seems to bounce up and down. When you ride in an automobile, your vision becomes unstable and road signs seem to vibrate or blur, becoming clear when you stop. The balance problem is worse in the dark, where you may stumble and fall.

Bilateral vestibular failure (BVF) occurs when the balance mechanism of both ears is damaged. By contrast, vertigo is a symptom of asymmetric, or one-sided, damage. BVF can occur with any disease that damages both ears, either one ear after the other or both ears at the same time. Most such diseases will also damage hearing, so any person who is deaf in both ears might have BVF. Some drugs and several genetic disorders can selectively damage the vestibular part of the inner ear and cause BVF without affecting hearing. Anyone who is taking drugs that may be toxic to vestibular function needs to know how to recognize early symptoms of damage so the drug can be stopped before the damage is severe.

The main symptoms of BVF are imbalance when standing and walking and visual distortion with head movement, called

oscillopsia. Since one of the main functions of the vestibular system is to keep the eyes stable when the head is moving, it is not surprising that after that system is damaged, the eyes move when the head moves and visual acuity is degraded. In order for a person with BVF to see clearly, she must stop and hold her head perfectly still. Some people with BVF find that they must hold their heads still with their hands on their chins in order to read.

BVF initially came to the attention of most doctors in the early 1940s, when a frequent treatment for Ménière's disease involved cutting the vestibular nerve. As noted in chapter 3, a small percentage of patients with Ménière's disease eventually develop disease in both ears—and in the past some patients had their vestibular nerves cut on both sides. After the second surgery, in which the vestibular nerve was cut on the side opposite to that of the first surgery, these patients had severe problems with balance and found their vision blurred when they were in motion. In some cases the symptoms of BVF were worse than the symptoms of Ménière's disease that surgery was intended to cure. For this reason, surgeons now rarely cut the vestibular nerve on both sides.

Awareness of BVF increased after streptomycin became widely used, around 1950, when it was one of the only treatments for tuberculosis. By then, tuberculosis had killed more than 1 billion people. But streptomycin can be extremely toxic to the vestibular system. After receiving streptomycin for suspected tuberculosis, a doctor named John Crawford described his symptoms in a famous 1952 letter to the editor of the *New England Journal of Medicine*, "Living without a balancing mechanism." He reported his feeling of imbalance to his doctors, but they disregarded the symptom and continued his streptomycin treatment. On his daily walks he had difficulty seeing the faces of passersby and developed the tactic of saying hello to everyone so as not to offend any friends he could not recognize. When contacted years later, when he was in his eighties, Dr. Crawford said that he still had the symptoms of BVF but had adapted and lived a reasonably normal life.

Streptomycin is now rarely used, but another antibiotic in the same class, gentamicin, is widely used and equally toxic to the vestibular system. It is remarkably selective for the vestibular system, which means that it affects that system but usually does not affect hearing. Gentamicin is an extremely popular drug for use in the hospital because it kills many different types of bacteria, and it is inexpensive. In some countries, such as China, it is one of the most commonly used antibiotics. While in the United States at least a hundred patients a year are recognized to develop BVF due to gentamicin toxicity, in China the number is likely in the thousands. Gentamicin is excreted by the kidneys, so it should not be given to patients with kidney failure, since even a single dose can cause BVF. Indeed, even in people without kidney failure, a single dose may be capable of causing BVF, but the risk is especially high if the kidneys are not able to eliminate the medication from the body at a normal rate. Other antibiotics in the same class (aminoglycosides), particularly tobramycin, can be vestibular toxic but are not nearly as selective to the vestibular system as gentamicin, which means that they also affect hearing. Another common aminoglycoside, vancomycin, and certain diuretic medications (water pills), notably furosemide (Lasix), do not on their own cause problems but instead increase the toxicity of gentamicin when given together with it or around the same time.

Any infectious disease that involves both ears can produce BVF. Bacterial meningitis, particularly in children, can spread to the inner ears and cause bilateral hearing loss and BVF. A very small percentage of people who have vestibular neuritis (see chapter 5) will have a recurrence on the opposite side, sometimes years after the initial episode. Autoimmune inner ear disease (AIED), either in isolation or in combination with systemic autoimmune diseases such as systemic lupus erythematosis (SLE) or rheumatoid arthritis, can cause BVF and bilateral hearing loss. Indeed, a significant proportion of people with BVF, whether from autoimmune disease or an infectious disease, may have a disease with an inflammatory component that might respond to treatment with anti-inflammatory corticosteroid medication or other immune-modulating medications. Some articles in the medical literature document people with BVF who have in their blood antibodies that bind to, and potentially adversely affect the function and health of, the inner ear balance system. Many of these people may not be harmed by these antibodies—that is, yes, there are antibodies, and yes, they bind to the inner ear, but no, these antibodies are not harmful to the inner ear. Nevertheless, this is an area in which there should be more research, especially since approximately half of the people with BVF appear to have a disease for which there is no known cause.

BVF can run in families, either as an isolated vestibular syndrome or as part of a more generalized neurological degenerative disorder. Several inherited spinocerebellar ataxias (SCAs) include BVF as a part of their profile. Genetic mutations that cause some of these disorders have been identified, but many have yet to be identified. Finally, there is a moderate decline in vestibular function with aging, similar to age-related hearing loss. However, full-blown BVF with severe imbalance and oscillopsia does not occur with normal aging.

Typical Symptoms of Bilateral Vestibular Failure

People with BVF have difficulty walking, especially in the dark or on uneven surfaces such as grass, dirt, or sand. They may have had bouts of vertigo in the past, but once BVF is near complete, the vertigo spells stop. When people with BVF view road signs from inside a moving vehicle, the letters seem to vibrate. The constant jiggling of the visual environment mostly stops when the car stops. Slight movements cause the visual environment to appear to jump around like a movie taken with a shaky camera. Over several years, people with BVF gradually improve as the brain learns to use other sensory information (primarily vision and the perception of position of various structures in the body—called proprioception) to replace the lost vestibular signals. However, the oscillopsia never completely resolves.

CASE EXAMPLE: Well but Wobbly

Brianna is a 25-year-old nurse with chronic kidney failure who was being treated with dialysis until she could receive a kidney transplant. She developed an infection of her dialysis shunt and was given a course of intravenous gentamicin because the bacteria cultured from the shunt were sensitive to gentamicin. Two days into the treatment she began noticing imbalance, particularly when she was in the shower washing her hair. She told her doctor, and he ordered a hearing test that came back normal. He told her that there was no sign of damage to the inner ears and that she should finish the ten-day course of gentamicin. Her balance became progressively worse and by the last few days of treatment she was having difficulty driving because she could not read road signs.

Her kidney specialist referred her to an ophthalmologist who told her that her eyes were fine and that she had normal visual acuity. She next saw a neurologist, who diagnosed Brianna with imbalance of unknown cause after an MRI of the brain was normal. Finally, she saw an ear specialist who ordered videonystagmography (VNG) and found absent response to caloric stimulation on both sides. Hearing tests were normal. The diagnosis of gentamicin ototoxicity was made, and she was told that there was relatively little that could be done except physical therapy for her balance.

Brianna's travails may seem extreme, but we have both seen similar cases in our practices. The medical system failed Brianna at several levels. First, her kidney specialist did not recognize that gentamicin is toxic to the vestibular system. He should not have given gentamicin to someone in kidney failure, and he should have been monitoring balance function rather than hearing while she was receiving the drug. Her ophthalmologist should have recognized that the problem was with eye stability during head movement. A simple eye test for BVF is the dynamic visual acuity (DVA) test. It is performed by having the patient read an eye chart with the head still and then read the chart while shaking the head back and forth at about two cycles per second. A drop in visual acuity of more than one line on the chart with head shaking suggests BVF. We recommend doing this test using a handheld card or paper designed to test close-up vision. Close-up vision with the head moving actually turns out to be more of a challenge to the balance system, compared to distance vision with the head moving. Finally, the neurologist could have recognized BVF by performing the head impulse test described in chapter 5. In Brianna's case there would be corrective eye movements after rapid head movements in both directions.

What Can I Do to Help My Doctor Make the Diagnosis?

The key is to recognize the symptom complex of imbalance and oscillopsia. You can easily test for oscillopsia by trying to read while shaking your head. It is normal to have a mild drop in visual clarity with head shaking. But if you cannot read at all with head shaking, you should alert your doctor. Also, if you receive intravenous antibiotics you should ask your doctor if it is one of the antibiotics that can damage the inner ear. If it is, both you and your doctor should be alert for symptoms of imbalance and oscillopsia.

What Laboratory Tests Should My Doctor Order and Why?

The symptoms of imbalance and oscillopsia are fairly easy to recognize, and a doctor can confirm the diagnosis using the dynamic visual acuity test described above and the head impulse test described in chapter 5. Both tests require some training but are easily learned. A definitive diagnosis requires videonystagmography or electronystagmography with caloric and rotational testing. Rotational testing is the gold standard, as caloric testing has technical limits and the results are less reliable than rotational testing. Unfortunately, rotational testing is usually only available at major medical centers. A quantitative video head impulse test using videonystagmography has recently been introduced and is becoming more generally available than rotational testing. Gentamicin and other antibiotic levels can and should be measured with blood tests. However, having levels within the target range does not guarantee that there will be no toxicity. Dizziness and balance-related symptoms and signs should still be monitored during treatment.

What Is the Best Treatment for BVF?

The mainstay of treatment for BVF is vestibular physical therapy with an experienced vestibular physical therapist. As much as possible, medications that suppress balance function and cause sedation should be avoided, as should additional courses of antibiotics that are toxic to the ear. In some cases of potentially life-threatening infections, such antibiotics are almost impossible to avoid, but in most people, for the majority of infections, other antibiotic options are available. If you have BVF, you have lost a major sensory system important for balance, and you need all other systems to function optimally. Therefore, if you have BVF, it is more important than ever to take care of your general health and vision.

As noted above, the possibility of autoimmune causes or inflammatory causes for unexplained BVF must be considered, particularly if there is associated hearing loss. Therefore, doctors often consider a trial of anti-inflammatory corticosteroid medications, colloquially referred to as "steroids." Steroids alarm doctors and their patients because of the potential for side effects. The challenge is to balance this fear against the potential to do good. Some doctors believe that no one should die without a trial of steroids. Thus, should we let inner ear cells die without a trial of steroids? At the same time, all experienced doctors have seen patients who have reacted badly to steroids; a very sick person treated with steroids might develop an overwhelming fungal infection or avascular necrosis of the hip that requires joint replacement surgery, or a perfectly healthy person might develop diabetes or transient psychosis. Short courses of steroids (one week) tend to be less risky than long courses (several weeks).

One question that often comes up is whether vestibular function lost in BVF might be replaced with a surgical implant.

You may know about the dramatic stories of people who were deaf but gained hearing from cochlear implants. In a cochlear implant system, a microphone picks up sound waves and converts them into electrical signals that are processed and ultimately fed into the cochlear nerve (or brain stem, in the case of the new auditory brain stem implants). The results of such artificial hearing systems are not identical to natural hearing, but it's a lot better than nothing.

Several academic centers are working on vestibular implants that would replace balance function in the same way that cochlear implants substitute for normal hearing function. The current concept is that a series of sensors would act similarly to the inner ear to detect both linear and angular accelerations of the head using linear and angular accelerometers. A computer would then translate this information into a code of electrical pulses transmitted to the vestibular nerve. For people with BVF who have not made an excellent recovery, the possibility of a vestibular prosthesis holds the promise to improve balance and stabilize vision. We are still several years out from large clinical trials to test a range of devices and protocols for treatment of BVF, but a few such devices have already been implanted, and preliminary results are encouraging.

What Can I Do on My Own to Treat BVF?

In addition to having a physical therapy program, you should continue with regular exercise as much as possible. Playing sports that involve balance and eye tracking, such as tennis and handball, are ideal. In many ways you should do the things that make you feel dizzy, since the brain needs to receive what physiologists call "error signals" to adapt to the vestibular loss. In other words, you need a signal that you are doing something wrong so that you can correct it. Fall prevention is a critical concern. It is important to keep some lights on at night because the imbalance is much worse in the dark. Be sure you can see where you are walking, and use railings. Finally, do not dive into deep water, because you may have difficulty telling which way is up and therefore are at risk for drowning.

Mimics of Bilateral Vestibular Failure

People with peripheral neuropathy (i.e., any disorder affecting the nerves of the arms and legs) have imbalance that is much worse in the dark, similar to people with BVF. However, people with peripheral neuropathy do not have oscillopsia, and they typically have numbness, tingling, or burning in the feet. Spinal cord diseases, most commonly compression of the spinal cord by herniated disks or calcified ridges inside the spinal canal, can lead to a prominent tendency to tip over, similar to what happens to people with BVF, though people with spinal cord compression do not have oscillopsia, and distinct spinal cord signs are visible to doctors when they do a physical examination. All diseases of the **cerebellum** can mimic BVF. People with cerebellar damage have both imbalance and oscillopsia but also typically have other findings, including poor coordination of the extremities, impaired visual tracking with the head still, or slurring of speech. As noted above, several inherited cerebellar ataxia disorders have a combination of cerebellar symptoms and BVF symptoms.

Red Flags
- Sudden onset of BVF and deafness. Consider treatment for occlusive vascular disease in the vertebrobasilar system (see chapter 6).

- Rapid onset of BVF and deafness over days to weeks (rather than years). Consider course of steroids for autoimmune disorder.
- Sensation of imbalance while receiving gentamicin. Consider the possibility that the drugs are toxic to the ears and stop ototoxic medications if possible.

CHAPTER 10

Small Vessel Ischemic Disease in the Deep White Matter

Over the past several years, you have been dizzy and off balance when you are on your feet and walking. You are much better sitting or lying down. The dizziness is difficult to describe, but it feels like your head is heavy. You need to hold on to railings more, and recently, you have started using a cane. Once you almost missed the chair when sitting down.

The brain has gray matter and white matter. The gray matter consists of dense clusters of neuronal cell bodies, while the **white matter** consists of bundles of neuronal fibers (axons) carrying information from neurons in one part of the brain to neurons in another. In fact, the gray matter, though enriched in neurons, actually has neuronal fibers running through it, and the white matter contains some neurons. Both the gray and white matter have supporting cells, called glia, that help provide nutrients to the neurons and fibers. Large regions of white matter are located in the center of the brain, around the fluid-filled spaces called the lateral ventricles. These regions deep in the center of the brain are known as the deep white matter of the brain, or the subcortical and periventricular white matter.

With the introduction of magnetic resonance imaging (MRI) techniques of the brain in the late 1970s, researchers observed that most normal older people showed changes in image intensity (**hyperintensity**) in the deep white matter. At first these so-called white matter hyperintensities seen on MRI were thought to be "normal aging phenomena," but with more research the amount of white matter hyperintensities was found to correlate with the degree of cognitive impairment and gait and balance dysfunction commonly seen in older people.

Why would deep white matter damage lead to dizziness and balance dysfunction? The neuronal fiber tracts running through the deep white matter, particularly those next to the lateral ventricles, carry motor signals from higher to lower brain centers important for gait and balance control, including what are called long loop postural reflexes. These reflexes carry sensory information from the legs, which travels to the brain for processing; then the brain sends motor signals all the way back down to the legs. Long loop reflexes are critical for maintaining upright posture and balance. People with damage to the periventricular white matter feel unsteady and are extremely susceptible to falls; some may fall heavily, "like a log," because their automatic corrective reflexes are not functioning.

The degree of white matter hyperintensities on MRI is a judgment call. Almost every older adult brain MRI we order has some bright signals in the deep white matter. In the 1990s such signals were referred to as unidentified bright objects (UBOs), a play on the phrase unidentified flying objects (UFOs), suggesting spacecraft from an alien world. Both UBOs and UFOs refer to observations that are controversial and of questionable significance. One has to wonder—if nearly every scan has these findings, how can they be abnormal? Our view is that abnormality in this case is a matter of degree. When large swaths of the white matter are very bright—we call this distribution "confluent"—we know with a high degree of confidence that something abnormal is occurring in the white matter.

Are there conditions other than aging that selectively involve the deep white matter of the brain? There's little doubt that long-term, uncontrolled hypertension and diabetes mellitus cause slow and steady accumulation of blockages in the small blood vessels of the brain. When these vessels become sufficiently occluded, a small area of the brain may suddenly be damaged in what is called a lacunar infarct or small stroke. Lacunar infarcts are common in the deep white matter, particularly in people with chronic hypertension and diabetes.

What happens if the narrowing of blood vessels is not sudden but instead gradually accumulates over the years? What if the narrowing does not totally prevent blood flow but instead chronically reduces blood flow below normal? We use the noncommittal term "narrowing" to describe this process, as there may be multiple common disease processes that narrow and occlude the small blood vessels supplying the deep white matter of the brain.

Blood flow reduction might not be so low as to cause symptoms that would bring a person to an emergency room. Nevertheless, some neurons and glial cells supplied by the narrowed blood vessels would likely become sick, and some might even die. One might call this situation chronic mild **ischemia**, meaning chronic impairment of blood flow of a sufficient magnitude to cause damage. The brain areas farthest from the heart, where blood pressure is the lowest (i.e., the deep white matter), would have the highest risk of injury due to low blood flow.

Deep brain blood flow is regulated by the small blood vessels supplying the white matter. This regulation is accomplished in part by smooth muscle cells that wrap around the small blood vessels and contract or relax to adjust the amount of blood received by each part of the brain, matching the flow of nutrients and oxygen to the activity of a particular region of the brain. If you are reading this book, the small blood vessels supplying your visual centers of the brain are dilated, allowing brain areas critical for vision to receive extra blood. If someone is reading this book to you, something similar is going on in the auditory—hearing-related—areas of the brain.

One disease that can affect brain blood flow is cerebral amyloid angiopathy (CAA). In CAA, an abnormal protein called amyloid is deposited in the walls of small blood vessels of the brain—the same protein that is deposited in the brain tissues in people who have **Alzheimer disease**. CAA can happen with or without accompanying Alzheimer disease. Aging is a major risk factor for both CAA and Alzheimer disease. Amyloid can narrow the small blood vessels and destroy their normal structure, including the smooth muscle cells important for blood flow regulation. Therefore, one would expect that someone affected with CAA would be unable to regulate brain blood flow normally and would be at an increased risk for brain injury related to low blood flow. In the 1990s we were among the first to point out a possible association between CAA and deep white matter abnormalities of the brain. We have also noted that some older people with imbalance of unknown cause, even if they don't have CAA, may have marked abnormal narrowing of small blood vessels of the brain, limiting blood flow. In short, any disease that disrupts the structure of small blood vessels of the brain creates a risk for chronic low brain blood flow. CAA is best known for its ability to cause rupture of blood vessels and large brain hemorrhages. However, when we look at the white matter on the MRI of people who have been diagnosed with CAA-related brain hemorrhage, we frequently see prominent abnormality of the deep white matter due to small vessel ischemic disease in addition to the hemorrhage.

Low blood flow to the brain from any cause, including impaired heart function, may lead to deep white matter damage and associated dizziness, imbalance, and abnormality of gait. People who have suffered a cardiac arrest, resulting in the sudden cessation of blood flow to the whole brain, may develop delayed degeneration of the deep white matter. The implication is that, whether sudden or gradual, widespread deep white matter ischemia (inadequate blood supply) in the brain may give rise to progressive deep white matter degeneration and deterioration of balance.

Atrial fibrillation is a heart rhythm abnormality or arrhythmia. One result of atrial fibrillation is that a less than normal amount of blood is pumped from the heart to the whole brain. This problem is especially serious when the heart rate is fast. If a person has atrial fibrillation and the heart rate is over 90, blood flow to the brain is usually impaired. We have seen a consistent association between atrial fibrillation, white matter abnormalities on brain MRI, and gait and balance symptoms.

Typical Symptoms of Chronic Decreased Blood Flow

The symptoms tend to be most prominent when standing and walking and least prominent when sitting or lying down. People describe a vague head sensation (anywhere from light-headed to heavy headed), but the main sensations are a feeling of unsteadiness and a fear of falling. People with chronic decreased blood flow lose their corrective reflexes, so when they fall, those falls can be devastating. Family members may note subtle changes in personality or cognition. These changes usually do not rise to the level of dementia, though sometimes they do, in which case the term "vascular dementia" is applied. For milder symptoms attributable to blood-flow-related damage in the brain, we use the term "vascular cognitive impairment."

CASE EXAMPLE: Is Aging a Disease?

Alfred is a 79-year-old retired judge who used to be physically fit. His only prior medical problem was hypertension, treated with various medications over the past 40 years. In recent years, he grabs on to furniture or walls or other people as he walks around. He feels fine when he is lying down. When sitting in a chair, he also feels close to normal but sometimes has a vague sense of "dizziness" in his head. When asked to describe the dizziness, he says, "There's just something wrong in my head." He has noted a mild decrease in his ability to multitask and to remember names. He fell last year when he caught his toe on a crack in the sidewalk and fractured his arm. He since has cut back on walking because of fear of falling.

Alfred's primary care doctor thought he might have a problem in the inner ear and referred him to an ear, nose, and throat specialist. The ENT doctor told him that his inner ears were fine and that he should see a neurologist. The neurologist noted that he had imbalance when walking and mild memory impairment but no sign of a stroke or other neurological disease. An MRI of the brain was read as showing "confluent areas of hyperintensity in the periventricular white matter representing small vessel ischemic disease commonly seen in patients of this age." The neurologist informed him that he was just getting older and had to accept the consequences.

Aging is not a disease. Although it is true that one must accept the consequences of aging, since there are no good alternatives, many of the diseases that commonly occur with aging can be successfully treated. Just because a condition occurs commonly with aging does not mean it is normal. In Alfred's case, the first line of treatment is to be sure he has adequate blood pressure to maintain perfusion of the area with small vessel disease in the deep white matter. Patients often are maintained on antihypertensive medications that they have been on for many years even though their blood pressure is on the low side. Alfred's diastolic pressure (lower number) should not be below 60 regardless of the systolic pressure (higher number), and a trial of antihypertensive medication may be warranted, just to see what happens to his symptoms. As with everything else in medicine, there is a fair amount of trial and error involved in getting the blood pressure right, and some of the interventions described in chapter 2 on orthostatic hypotension may come into play in scenarios similar to this. The second line of treatment should be a physical therapy program aimed at gait and balance training and strengthening exercises. People with balance problems often cut back on activities, as Alfred did, which leads to weakness in the legs further aggravating the balance problem (a classic vicious cycle).

What Can I Do to Help My Doctor Make the Diagnosis?

If you have had a chronic balance problem that remains unexplained, you must communicate this to your doctor. If you do not speak up and characterize your balance symptoms as a problem, your doctor may not recognize that there is anything out of the ordinary. In some cases, in the hustle and bustle of a busy medical office, gait may not be examined. If you feel you have a balance problem, and your doctor has not checked out how you walk, a ten-second demonstration of walking around an exam room is usually more than sufficient to see that there is a problem. Your doctor may indeed want to try physical therapy, to see if you get better, before embarking on an elaborate diagnostic work-up, and this may be fine. However, if your problems persist despite a trial of physical therapy, and if the diagnosis remains unknown, it may be time to consult with a specialist.

What Laboratory Tests Should My Doctor Order and Why?

The tests most likely to reveal a diagnosis in people with small vessel disease of the deep white matter is a brain MRI or CT and potentially tests of heart function such as a Holter monitor or echocardiogram. Because of the extremely high prevalence of various blood flow problems, there is no doubt that additional blood-flow-related tests will in the future be used to better assess people who have the problems discussed in this chapter. To give one example, the same tests that are being developed for identification of amyloid in the brains of people with Alzheimer disease may one day be used to identify CAA without Alzheimer disease. Currently CAA is diagnosed based on the presence of hemorrhages in the brain, but this may be just the tip of the iceberg.

What Is the Best Treatment for Small Vessel Disease of the Deep White Matter?

One answer is to improve blood flow to the brain where possible. Improving blood flow to the brain is a project that spans multiple medical specialties, including but not limited to cardiology and neurology. You may have multiple cardiovascular issues that need attention. Simple measures such as stopping a medication that is lowering blood pressure or causing sedation or starting a medication to improve heart function may be helpful. As in the case example described above, physical therapy should always be considered. Regular exercise improves circulation throughout the body, including the brain.

Is it possible to repair the areas of the brain that have already been damaged by small vessel ischemic disease? The short is answer is no, but a longer answer is that this may be possible in the future. Recent insights obtained from research using stem cells to treat cerebral palsy may be applicable to this problem. Cerebral palsy is a common cause of disability in children, often in children born prematurely. Impaired blood flow to the brain results in damage and impaired development throughout the brain but particularly in the white matter.

In the white matter, there is a class of glial cells, called oligodendrocytes, that are damaged by low blood flow. Oligodendrocytes wrap around the long nerve fibers (axons) of neurons that run through the deep white matter. Oligodendrocytes produce a protein called myelin, which acts as an insulator for the nerve fibers and is critical for normal transmission of signals through the fibers. Without oligodendrocytes, there would be no myelin in the brain. And without myelin, the circuits of the brain would not work. A stark example is multiple sclerosis, a demyelinating disease in which the myelin is damaged by inflammation. Signals can move along demyelinated nerves but at a markedly reduced speed, resulting in loss of function.

Studies of oligodendrocytes suggest that these cells might play a role in treatment of white matter disorders. Researchers in the United States and Germany have begun to use stem cells obtained from umbilical cord blood as a treatment for cerebral palsy in children. After intravenous infusion, stem cells have the capacity to travel to the injured white matter, deep in the brain, and facilitate repair. Under appropriate conditions stem cells can develop into—that is, differentiate into—oligodendrocytes. Could the use of cord-blood-derived stem cells potentially be extended to adults with white matter disease who have dizziness and imbalance? We do not yet know. That it works in children doesn't necessarily mean that it would work in adults; the infant brain is more plastic than the adult brain.

Do stem cells exist in the deep white matter of the adult brain? Recent research suggests that indeed there are immature cells in the white matter of adults that in some ways resemble the stem cells of umbilical cord blood. These cells, which one might loosely call stem cells, are present throughout life, though their functions have not yet been fully clarified. One example is a type of immature oligodendrocyte, called the oligodendrocyte precursor cell (OPCs). These cells are widespread in the adult central nervous system. In the normal brain, they appear to have something to do with maintaining the integrity of myelin. Might OPCs and other similar cells somehow be activated and encouraged to participate in white matter repair? This remains to be determined. Several research labs are working on ways to encourage OPCs to develop into mature oligodendrocytes.

What Can I Do on My Own to Treat Small Vessel Disease of the Deep White Matter?

The main focus should be on exercise and physical retraining; start by working with a physical therapist on your balance and walking. Try to find a physical therapist with an interest in balance disorders (some PTs are specialized in other areas and would not be appropriate for you). Ask the physical therapist to design a home exercise program that you can use, on your own, to extend the benefits of physical therapy.

Sip on fluids that do not contain caffeine—such as water—throughout the day, and ask your doctor what is the maximum amount of fluid per day that you can safely consume. Some people need to limit water intake, notably those with congestive heart failure. Review your medication list with your doctor, as some medications have the potential to interfere with brain function. It is usually a good idea to take the lowest effective dose of medication because all medications have side effects, and side effects tend to be more evident at higher doses.

Get an automatic blood-pressure cuff to track your blood pressure and heart rate at home. If your symptoms are most prominent when you are standing up, don't forget to take some readings while you are having symptoms standing up. This may seem obvious, but people, including doctors, routinely measure blood pressure and heart rate in the sitting position, even though the symptoms occur when standing up. This information may indicate to your doctors whether you have low blood pressure or high or low heart rates, all of which relate to brain blood flow. As with all balance disorders, it may be beneficial to see an ophthalmologist or optometrist and optimize your vision, which helps with normal balance and walking and reduces the risk of falls.

Mimics of Small Vessel Ischemic Disease in the Deep White Matter

The gait disorder of **Parkinson disease** can mimic that of small vessel ischemic disease in the deep white matter. Both can have a shuffling quality, and people with both disorders tend to take turns slowly and carefully. However, most people with Parkinson disease have many other features, including tremor, muscle rigidity, and lack of facial expression that are not typically seen with small vessel ischemic disease.

Hydrocephalus exerts pressure on the periventricular white matter and produces a gait disorder very much like that of small vessel ischemic disease of the white matter. MRI of the brain can usually easily distinguish between these two disorders, although sometimes it can be difficult to distinguish enlarged ventricles (ventriculomegaly) caused by increased pressure from that due to atrophy of the surrounding white matter.

Cervical spinal stenosis caused by arthritic and disk disorders of the cervical spine can lead to a slow compression of the spinal cord, producing a slowly progressive gait disorder with leg weakness, but invariably a neurological examination will discover other symptoms of spinal stenosis, including spasticity of the legs. In addition, many people with spinal cord compression have urinary urgency or incontinence.

People with Alzheimer disease and other degenerative causes of dementia can have mild gait impairment related in part to weakness and lack of activity, but the degree of cognitive impairment is much greater and earlier in onset than the balance impairment.

Red Flags
- Sudden worsening of symptoms. This may suggest a stroke due to large vessel occlusion.
- Numbness or weakness of one or both legs; urinary urgency or incontinence. The person should be examined for spinal cord damage, also known as myelopathy.
- Tremor of the hands and slowness of movement. Parkinson disease or another related neurodegenerative disorder may be the cause.

- Cognitive impairment and urinary incontinence. Normal pressure hydrocephalus (NPH) may be the cause.
- Major loss of cognitive function. Alzheimer disease and other types of dementia may be the cause.

Acknowledgments

We would like to express our gratitude to Jacqueline Wehmueller and all the others at Johns Hopkins University Press who understood the value of a book about dizziness. Dr. Whitman would like to thank his wife, Sally, and the rest of his family who encouraged and supported the writing of this book, including his children, Cole and Jalisa, and his parents, Steven and Sheila; Thomas Sabin, for teaching so many of us best practices in neurology; and Steven Rauch, Richard Lewis, and many others in otolaryngology at Massachusetts Eye and Ear who have found time to discuss the vestibular system and approaches to the treatment of dizziness. Dr. Baloh would like to thank his wife, Grace, and children, Bob and Nicole, for providing inspiration; Vicente Honrubia, John Mazziotta, and the many other colleagues in head and neck surgery and neurology at UCLA Health, who over the years provided support and encouragement; and his many fellows and trainees, who provided the need to learn and discover.

Appendix

Home Exercises

Exercises for people with impaired balance may be divided into two types: exercises intended to improve gait and balance for everyone, regardless of the problem, and exercises specifically designed to retrain how the ear and brain work together.

The two general goals of a balance exercise program are, first, improving mobility and, second, preventing falls. A balance exercise program should include exercises focused on:

- Ability to control your body position and distribution of weight in space, sometimes described as your center of mass.
- Strength, particularly in the thighs and legs, so that if you do lose your balance, you will have more power to recover.
- Range of motion of joints, including the shoulders, hips, knees, and ankles.
- Cardiovascular function.

To improve strength, practice standing up from a chair. If you have access to a gym, supervised pool, or community center that has balance or strength-training classes, consider taking advantage of these valuable resources.

Exercises that address all of the above goals can be found on the National Institutes of Health (NIH) website. Search within the web pages associated within the various institutes of the NIH, using as a search term any of the disorders discussed in this book. For example, an excellent site called Go4Life from the National Institute on Aging includes useful videos and explains and describes exercises addressing the four areas of focus listed above (https://go4life.nia.nih.gov /exercises).

People who have suffered a loss of vestibular function in the ear or vestibular nerve have specific needs. The brain needs to be challenged to analyze motion even though it is receiving faulty information from one ear. This is accomplished in medical practice with some variation of vestibular exercises that include

- Tracking visual targets with head still, then with head moving.
- Rapid head movements when sitting, then walking.
- Walking in the dark and on uneven surfaces.

Instructions for performing vestibular exercises can be found at www .dizziness-and-balance.com/treatment/rehab/cawthorne.html.

We are often asked how long after an inner ear injury a person must continue exercises. We find that people usually know when it is all right for them to discontinue these exercises. If you stop doing home exercises too soon—that is, before your brain has compensated fully for your inner ear problem—you may note a recurrence of dizziness or imbalance that once again improves when you resume exercises. The typical reasonable range of duration for an exercise program after an episode of vestibular neuritis or labyrinthitis is weeks to months.

For people who have not been diagnosed with a loss of vestibular function, it is still beneficial to do exercises aimed at improving balance, strength, range of motion, and cardiovascular fitness.

Walking on uneven ground, such as grass, dirt, or sand, is an excellent challenge for balance. If it can be done safely—without a significant risk of falling—walking on uneven ground usually helps people improve their balance. Tai chi and qigong are ancient arts that train balance. Classes are available in many communities, and videos may be found on the web. Many community centers, senior centers, and recreation centers also host free or inexpensive balance classes led by local physical therapists.

If you are having difficulty walking, or can only walk a short distance before getting tired, it may be beneficial to see a neurologist who can analyze your walking difficulty and potentially identify specific abnormalities. For walking to occur normally, a symphony of movements must happen just right. If anything is off just a little, the person may become exhausted when walking some distance and may have an increased risk of falls. For example, if your foot doesn't clear the floor easily, or if your muscles aren't strong enough to pick your thigh up at the hip, you may be expending an unnecessary amount of energy with each step.

Many physical therapists are adept at figuring out what exactly is not working well functionally, though they often appreciate some input from a neurologist to help guide design of an individualized treatment plan. If you see a physical therapist, work with him or her to start an individualized home exercise plan as early as possible in the course of your treatment.

Glossary

anxiety A negative emotion experienced in anticipation of a real or imagined threat.

autoimmune inner ear disease Illness in which one's own immune system attacks the inner ear causing hearing loss with or without vertigo, and which responds to immunosuppressive medication such as prednisone.

autoimmune neuropathy A collection of disorders in which one's own immune system attacks and injures the nerves including those of the arms and legs.

benign paroxysmal positional vertigo (BPPV) Common cause of vertigo resulting from debris in a semicircular canal (usually the posterior), manifested by brief bouts of vertigo and nystagmus with position change.

brain tumor An abnormal growth of cells in the brain that can compress surrounding normal brain.

canalithiasis The most common variant of benign paroxysmal positional vertigo (BPPV), in which otoconia (defined below) are free floating within the semicircular canal.

canalith repositioning maneuvers Treatments intended to move displaced otoconia from the affected semicircular canal to the utricle. An example is the Epley maneuver (defined below).

cells Biological building blocks, out of which are made tissues, organs, and ultimately whole organisms.

central nervous system (CNS) The brain and spinal cord.

central positional vertigo A rare situation in which a brain disorder causes positional vertigo.

central vestibular pathways Pathways in the brain carrying vestibular signals.

cerebellum Portion of the back of the brain that modulates balance, limb coordination, eye movements, and, to some extent, cognition.

cervical spinal stenosis Narrowing of the normal fluid filled space around the spinal cord in the neck.

CT scan A computed tomography (from Greek *tomos*, meaning cut or slice) scan, a set of technologies using x-rays to create images of the body resembling slices of a loaf of bread or to reconstruct such slices into a 3D image.

diabetic neuropathy Deterioration of the sensory, motor, and, in some cases, autonomic nerves resulting in a clinical syndrome that may involve weakness, numbness, tingling, and burning.

differential diagnosis The list of diagnoses possible to explain a symptom or cluster of symptoms. A doctor makes a differential diagnosis when considering explanations for a patient's symptoms.

disequilibrium Inability to maintain normal balance, leading to a risk for falls.

diuretic A class of medication that causes the kidney to increase the amount of fluids and electrolytes removed from the blood.

Dix-Hallpike test Test for the posterior semicircular variant of benign paroxysmal positional vertigo (BPPV).

dizziness Any abnormal head sensation, including vertigo, lightheadedness, faintness, imbalance, and spatial disorientation.

embolic Type of stroke caused by pieces of clot originating from the heart or large arteries traveling downstream to eventually block smaller blood vessels.

endolymph Fluid inside the membranous labyrinth of the inner ear.

epileptic seizures and/or epilepsy Recurrent, unprovoked disturbances of brain function caused by abnormal synchronized activity of many neurons in the brain.

Epley maneuver Commonly used canalith repositioning maneuver (defined above) for treating the posterior semicircular canal variant of benign paroxysmal positional vertigo (BPPV).

external ear The earlobe, or pinna (from Latin word for wing), plus the external ear canal, where a doctor can look with an otoscope. The inner boundary of the external ear is the eardrum, also known as the tympanic membrane.

glial cells Non-neuron cells (e.g., oligodendrocytes, astrocytes, and microglial cells) found in the human nervous system, all of which support and regulate the normal function of neurons.

gravitational field A collection of points in space, and the value at each point of the force per unit mass experienced by matter, as a result of being close to other matter. On Earth the acceleration due to gravity at sea level is 9.8 meters per second squared.

hydrocephalus Enlargement of the normal fluid-filled spaces inside the brain called ventricles.

hydrops Distention of the endolymphatic space (see endolymph defined above) within the membranous labyrinth. This finding is currently found in a postmortem, but potentially in the future it will be an MRI finding commonly seen in people with Ménière's disease (defined below).

hyperintensity A bright area on an MRI scan.

imbalance A synonym for disequilibrium (defined above).

inner ear Also known as the labyrinth. A portion of the ear deep in the skull that includes the balance organs (semicircular canals and otolith organs) and hearing organ (cochlea).

ischemia Decreased blood flow that is sufficiently low to present a substantial risk of damage to tissues, including but not limited to nervous system tissues such the brain and spinal cord.

labyrinth The inner ear, including the cochlea and vestibular organs.

labyrinthitis Inflammation of the inner ear (believed usually to be due to a viral infection) causing vertigo and hearing loss.

mal de debarquement syndrome (MdDS) A constant feeling of rocking and imbalance, usually after exposure to certain types of motion, such as on a boat, automobile, or airplane.

Ménière's disease A disorder of unknown cause that results in prolonged attacks of vertigo, typically lasting hours, and asymmetrical hearing loss that involves the hearing for low pitched sounds. Sometimes used synonymously with the term "endolymphatic hydrops," though studies suggest that a person can have Ménière's disease without endolymphatic hydrops, and vice versa.

middle ear The middle portion of the ear between the eardrum and inner ear, where tiny bones known as ossicles—the malleus (hammer), incus (anvil), and stapes (stirrup)—conduct sound from the outside world to the oval window, introducing sound waves into the inner ear.

migraine A genetically determined, electrical and chemical disorder of the brain that involves headache associated with nausea and/or excessive sensitivity to light (photophobia) but also many other symptoms, including excessive sensitivity to visual and physical motion and many types of dizziness.

migraine with aura Migraine headache with associated neurological symptoms such as weakness, numbness, loss and distortion of vision, and slurred speech.

motion sickness A syndrome of dizziness, perspiration, nausea, vomiting, increased salivation, yawning, and generalized malaise induced by motion (e.g., of a car, bus, airplane, or ship).

MRI scan Magnetic resonance imaging scan, a set of technologies that uses no x-rays but instead employs a powerful magnet and radio waves to make high resolution images of the body.

multiple sclerosis An autoimmune disorder of the brain and spinal cord resulting in multiple areas of damage to the cerebral white matter separated in space and time.

multiple system atrophy A degenerative brain disease of unknown cause that results in slow loss of numerous neurological functions, including but not limited to gait and balance function.

neuron A type of human nervous system cell that communicates with other similar cells through a combination of electrical and chemical processes.

nystagmus A rhythmic, repetitive jerking of the eyes with alternating slow phases, in which the eyes drift in one direction, and fast phases, in which the eyes jerk in the opposite direction.

orthostatic hypotension A sustained drop in blood pressure while sitting or standing, of a sufficient magnitude to adversely influence blood flow to the brain.

oscillopsia Instability of the visual scene with head movement, as while riding in a moving vehicle or walking, usually due to a failure of the semicircular canal–ocular reflexes.

otoconia Calcium carbonate containing crystals mixed with protein and embedded within the membranes that overlie the otolith organs (utricle and saccule).

otolith organs Organs within the inner ear that sense linear acceleration, including gravity.

Parkinson disease A brain disorder, resulting in slowing of movement, tremor, shuffling gait and other symptoms, many of which respond favorably to treatment with the medication levodopa.

peripheral vestibular system The balance-related portions of the inner ear (semicircular canals and otolith organs) plus the vestibular nerve, which connects the inner ear to the brain.

pheochromocytoma A rare tumor of the adrenal gland that secretes epinephrine and norepinephrine, causing attacks of dizziness, high blood pressure and fast heart rate, usually diagnosed with urine tests and/or MRI of the abdomen.

physiology The study of how living organisms or parts of the body function.

postural orthostatic tachycardia syndrome (POTS) A sustained rise in heart rate of at least 30–40 beats per minute that occurs when a person stands in one place for 10 minutes or less resulting in dizziness and other neurological symptoms.

rotational vertebral artery syndrome A rare syndrome in which turning the head compresses a vertebral artery, in its course through the neck, leading to compromised blood flow to portions of the brain stem and/or cerebellum.

saccule A chamber of the inner ear that contains one of the two otolith organs for sensing linear acceleration.

semicircular canals Circular tubes in the inner ear that sense angular acceleration.

specificity With respect to a physical finding on examination or diagnostic test, specificity measures how often the test or finding will correctly identify normal people as normal. A finding with a low specificity is often called a nonspecific finding.

stroke A brain attack, in which parts of the brain are damaged by either blockage of blood flow or hemorrhage.

syncope A transient loss of consciousness, typically due to a drop in blood flow to the whole brain.

thrombotic Of or pertaining to thrombosis, in which a blood clot forms within a blood vessel.

transient ischemic attack (TIA) A temporary and critical decrease in the amount of blood flow in one or a small set of blood vessels in the brain, resulting in brain-related symptoms that resolve within a few minutes to hours.

utricle Chamber of the inner ear that contains one of two otolith organs. It is the chamber where loose otoconia settle after treatment of benign paroxysmal positional vertigo (BPPV).

vasovagal syncope A form of syncope (defined above) that occurs in the setting of abnormal nervous system reflexes, characteristically involving an inappropriate slowing of the heart rate. Often used synonymously with the term "neurocardiogenic syncope."

vertebrobasilar Of or pertaining to one or both of the vertebral arteries and/or the basilar artery in the back of the brain, all of which are important for blood supply to the brain stem and cerebellum.

vertigo A false sense that the environment is moving (usually rotating) when it is stationary, or by some definitions, also a false sense of self-motion.

vestibular migraine A disorder in which migraine causes dizziness, sometimes even when the affected person does not have a headache.

vestibular neuritis Also known as vestibular neuronitis. Inflammation of the vestibular nerve (believed to be usually viral) causing severe vertigo and imbalance (with normal hearing) with improvement of vertigo over days, and improvement of balance over weeks to months.

vestibular schwannoma Benign tumor, also known as an acoustic neuroma, that usually originates from the vestibular nerve and typically manifests with a one-sided hearing loss.

vestibular system A set of anatomical structures and systems that includes the inner ear balance organs, the vestibular nerve from the ear to the brain, and the connections of the vestibular nerve in the brain, including but not limited to the vestibular nuclei in the brain stem.

videonystagmography (VNG) A method of eye movement recording in which a camera visualizes one or both eyes while a computer tracks and records eye movements during a variety of balance tests.

white matter Bundles of nerve fibers within the brain and spinal cord carrying signals from one part of the nervous system to another.

Index